The
TOXICOLOGY
Of
Botanical
MEDICINES

The TOXICOLOGY *Of* *Botanical* MEDICINES

Third Edition

Francis Brinker, N.D.

Eclectic Medical Publications,
Sandy, Oregon

In all cases of poisoning the local Poison Control Center should be contacted immediately for information and instructions before any intervention is attempted, other than removing the source of poison from the victim. If the number of such a center cannot be located, call a hospital, physician, or pharmacist for instructions. If a phone is not available, transport the victim to the nearest medical treatment facility and if possible bring the poisonous substance along for positive identification.

Permissions

Eclectic Medical Publications

36350 SE Industrial Way,

Sandy, OR 97055

Printed in the USA

ISBN 1-888483-09-1 paperback.

Library of Congress Catalog Card Number: 99 85790

Editorial and Production by Nancy Stodart

Book and Cover Design, Composition by Richard Stodart

Acknowledgements

I would especially like to thank the late Wade Boyle, N.D., for his extensive help in preparing the original manuscript. Also helpful with suggestions and encouragement at that time were Ed Alstat, N.D., Ed Hofman-Smith, N.D., and Stephen Sporn, N.D

The Oregon Poison Control And Drug Information Center at the University of Oregon's Health Science Center deserves special thanks for graciously allowing me to use their database on plant toxicities.

Contents

Preface To The Third Edition

As more pharmocological and clinical data on medicinal plants becomes available, the toxicology of these agents grows increasingly more refined. The number of literature references has been greatly increased in this edition to provide an updated review of this expansive topic.

Revisions have been made to further clarify vital information. Botanical nomenclature has been expanded to facilitate identification through scientific taxonomy and common English-language names. Doses are now listed in metric units, often with their English equivalents as well. Sundry notes are included which provide information that is pertinent for particular plants. If the toxic effects listed are primarily produced by a particular fraction or isolated constituent, this has been noted. (An appendix has also been added to furnish information on nontoxic plants that provide potentially toxic distilled volatile oil fractions that are commonly used as essential oils.) Signs and symptoms of toxity have been listed in the appropriate order of their chronological appearance. Treatments include both traditional and modern techniques and are differentiated as immediate first aid, additional medical intervention, and other adjunctive approaches.

While various treatment options are listed, this text does not provide in-depth instructions for managing cases of accidental plant poisonings or medicinal overdoses. The information provided here is primarily intended to serve as a quick reference for preventing or assessing adverse effects from botanical substances.

Francis J. Brinker, N.D.
November 4, 1999

Introduction

My hope in beginning this project was to produce a concise compilation of past and up-to-date information on the toxic effects of plants and plant extracts used medicinally by naturopathic physicians and taught at naturopathic colleges. The need for such a reference text does not stem from aggressive prescribing by our physicians; any dosages producing toxic manifestations are far in excess of naturopathic prescriptions, which are often fractional or attenuated for the most potent plants. Rather, the growing popularity of herbs and the consequent dangers of unwarranted use (either contraindicated applications or excessive dosage) among those who are poorly informed on herb collection or the home prescribing of potent herbs make reference texts on these topics necessary. Accidental poisoning in children and misidentification of poisonous plants as safe herbs that are similar in appearance also occur. It is not uncommon to receive calls at naturopathic clinics regarding possible side effects from herb use. A ready reference on this information should at all times be available.

The information presented in this text reviews the toxicology of medicinal plants as noted in pharmacology, pharmacognosy and botanical medicine texts used in former courses at the National College of Naturopathic Medicine (NCNM) and updated with recent publications and articles from medical journals. Accurate application of this information to cases of accidental poisoning can only be made when positive identification of the plant or its extract is made by a physician knowledgeable in pharmacognosy. Botanists, herbalists or florists may be of assistance in this regard.

This study is in no way intended to impugn skillful herbal practitioners or scare the lay public into indiscriminately avoiding the use of herbs. Botanicals are successfully used as sources of physiological nutritive complexes and pharmacologically active compounds, but, as with other foods and drugs, excessive or prolonged use can produce undesirable effects or unnecessary dependencies. Therefore, certain potent plants should be used only under the supervision of physicians educated in their pharmacologic and toxicologic qualities.

The use of commercially available herbs in general is quite safe. The first and sometimes only symptom of overdose is gastroenteritis. This results in vomiting and diarrhea which serve to expel the substance and thereby prevent excessive absorption. Quite often the toxic side effects are due to only one of the many active substances found in the plant. When isolated, the toxic compound may be potentially dangerous in minute amounts. Together with the other components of crude plant part or its extract, however, its toxic effects are often modified. This can significantly alter the pure drug effect and larger amounts of the toxic substance may be tolerated.

Concentration of particular toxic compounds differ from one herb product to another due to variations in factors affecting growth, processing, and storage. The variable absorption from different forms, the routes of administration, and individual patient sensitivity or idiosyncratic response to potent compounds also contribute to the uncertainty of adverse effects being produced. Therefore, it is important for the practitioner to be familiar not only with common therapeutic dosage ranges but also with the toxic side effects that can occur from whole herbs, their extracts, and their components. With products containing concentrated active constituents, the increased potency further necessitates accurate dosing.

People too often underestimate the potential for adverse effects from excessive doses of natural products such as herbs ("If a little is good, a lot is better"). Obviously, clear instructions for use (for example, "shake well before using," or "for external use only") and dose (for example, "ten drops three times each day before meals," and not "as needed") are of paramount importance in prescribing potent herbs and in preventing any danger arising from a potentially tragic misunderstanding of their power. The consequence of simply not shaking a bottle of liquid extract in which potent components may have precipitated and settled on the bottom can lead to the concentration in the last few doses and an overdose of that component while staying within the normal dosage range of the liquid extract. For this reason, since alkaloids are precipitated by tannins or salicylates, these mixtures should be avoided in prescriptions to prevent alkaloidal concentration in the bottom of the dispensing container.

Patients should be warned explicitly about the toxic potential of botanical substances for which this is an issue, since many assume that herbs are completely benign. Patients should also be assured that the use of powerful botanical agents in naturopathic practice has always followed the precept that minimum dosage is the most effective means to positively influence function or synergize innocuous substances. "Primum non nocere" (First, do no harm) is the philosophy of naturopathic botanical medicine, as in all its modalities.

By no means does this work pretend to be comprehensive in either its listing of toxic plants or in the information regarding those chosen for inclusion. What it does provide is the essential information for a basic knowledge of human reactions to certain plant toxins. Sharing this information to either prevent consumption of a toxic excess or assist a person following ingestion of a plant toxin will be a valuable service of naturopathic physicians to their community.

Recognizing the limitations resulting from my approach, I nevertheless feel the information contained herein will be useful to doctors and serious students of botanical medicine who wish to practice their art in a safe and successful manner.

Explanation of Format

Names: Scientific, Family and Common Names

The plants selected include many that may be used by naturopathic physicians, those available through personal collection or cultivation, and/or others that are available commercially to the public at large. The list of potentially toxic botanical substances that makes up the main text of this work is ordered alphabetically according to the scientific binomial names for the herbs. In a few cases, where many species in a genus may be used interchangeably, only the genus is identified. Several species of the same genus are grouped together if they have toxic constituents in common. Where scientific names have been recently changed or are still used interchangeably by some, the alternate name is given in parentheses following an = sign. The family name for each herb is added to help associate similar chemical effects or individual sensitivity to a larger group of related plants. Since many common names exist for each herb and several herbs can share the same common name, less emphasis is placed on this term for purposes of proper identification. However, the first listed common name is usually the most familiar and is typically used in literature references.

Two species formerly considered plants and included in my materia medica references as such, are not currently classified as members of the plant kingdom. *Amanita muscaria* and *Claviceps purpurea* are fungus, now grouped in the protist kingdom with bacteria, algae, molds and protozoa. Since the time of reclassification, many other fungus and protists have been found to contain medicinal activity, including *Penicillium* spp. of molds and *Streptomyces* spp. of bacteria. These organisms have not been included in this text due to their former lack of common use as remedies and based on their current status, even though they include substances now commonly used that have known toxicities (for example, griseofulvin/penicillin and erythromycin/tetracycline from the above genera, respectively).

Parts Containing Toxins:

Toxic Constituents

Because constituents and their concentrations can vary widely within a plant, the part of the plant used must be known in order to evaluate a reaction to a botanical substance. Certain plants are included, though their common use as crude herbs is innocuous, if commercially available extracts are sufficiently concentrated to be potentially hazardous (for example, essential oils of culinary/medicinal herbs and spices) or if some other part of the plant is toxic (for example, the whole bean of the Castor plant from which the oil is extracted).

The toxic constituents listed may or may not be the chief active medicinal component. Since constituents are generally more toxic when isolated and purified, their side effects can be minimized by using simple (crude) herb preparations. Concentration ranges for constituents are listed when known.

The toxicity of that constituent when used alone does not exactly describe the toxicity of the plant. For example, more of the active toxic component may be tolerated when it is in its natural complex equilibrium with other components. However, the known toxic dose and symptomology for a specific component can be extrapolated according to its concentration in the whole plant to suggest potential problems and management protocol for the intact plant or its extracts. The chemical class of the isolated toxic substance is noted to indicate probable solubility in different solvents and for comparison to other plants containing similar components.

Doses: Therapeutic, Toxic and Lethal

When known, toxic and fatal doses are noted according to the form of the substance consumed, as indicated. When doses are given as "/kg" this infers by body weight in kilograms (conversion from pounds given below). The normal therapeutic dose for a 70 kg (155 pound) adult is typically presented to give an appreciation for the relative power of the herb or its various preparations in several forms for comparisons sake, according to the information available from the references. The maximum amount in a therapeutic dosage range should not be exceeded without good reason, and the initial dose should always be less than the maximum recommended. The usual frequency for taking the therapeutic dosage can be assumed to be three times daily unless otherwise noted.

In specifying units of volume, previously used household

terms (for example, teaspoons and ounces) and apothecary terminology (for example, drams and grains) are now described in metric terminology (for example, milliliters and milligrams) for the sake of consistency, based on the following table. Universal agreement on the conversion of some household measurements to metric equivalents is lacking. I have used as a standard the source which defined these measurements for American medicine plants in the early part of the twentieth century, the *United States Pharmacopeia* IX of 1916, since much of the knowledge about botanical toxicology and toxic doses in humans was developed in that period through clinical experience with medicinal plants. These same equivalencies were specified in Felter's *Eclectic Materia Medica* in 1922 (ref. #9), the culmination of American Eclectic medical knowledge on plants.

Some household terms have been retained, particularly the term 'drops' when small doses are described, since these are still quite commonly used in describing doses. **The designation of a drop as used in this text refers to a specific liquid dosage based on the scientifically measured volume of a drop of water (called a minim).** Alcohol is less cohesive than water, so one drop of 50% alcoholic tincture is about one half of one minim. For this reason milliliters are the preferred dosage unit for accurately measuring liquids. **The more accurate milliliter equivalents of the drop (minim) doses are also given in this text.** One standard drop is equivalent to 0.06 ml, derived from 16.2 drops per milliliter. The exception to the following standard equivalencies for this text is the drop volume for essential oils, based on their unique and consistently smaller size and behavior. A drop in reference to essential or volatile oils in Appendix A is equivalent to 0.05 ml, 20 drops per milliliter. Based on the older sources of herbal and clinical toxicity which employed the household or apothecary systems of weights and measures, the following are the equivalencies used for converting doses within and between these and the metric system and the abbreviations used in the text.

Liquid volume:

> one minim (M) = one drop water
>
> one milliliter (ml) = 16.2 minims = 1000 microliters (mcl)
>
> one fluid dram (dr) = 60 minims = 3.7 milliliters
>
> one teaspoon (tsp) = one fluid dram = 0.125 fluid ounce
>
> one fluid ounce (oz) = 29.6 milliliter

Dry weight:

> one grain (gr) = 64.8 milligrams (mg)
>
> one gram (gm) = 15.4 grains
>
> one ounce (oz) = 480 grains = 31.1 grams
>
> one kilogram (kg) = 2.2 pounds (lb)

In describing the different types or forms of liquid extracts, the concentration can be inferred according to the type of extract identified. Fluid extracts are made with a weight to volume ratio of 1:1, for instance, one gram of dried plant material per one milliliter of liquid extract. For tinctures of potent botanical drugs the ratio is 1:10, that is, ten grams of plant material to 100 milliliters of extract. Most other tinctures not regulated as drugs are described as the traditional potency weight to volume ratio of 1:5, that is, twenty grams of plant substance is represented by 100 milliliter of extract. Many modern liquid botanical extracts sold commercially may be in a ratio from 1:5 to 1:1. Doses will vary accordingly. A hydroalcoholic solvent, that is, a mixture of water and ethanol, is used to make fluid extracts and tinctures. The proportions of ethanol to water vary depending on the constituents that are being extracted. To effectively extract and maintain particular components in solution, the alcohol content must be varied according to chemical nature of the desired constituent. In general the typical alcohol concentration to maximize extraction and maintain solubility is 90% for resins, 60-70% for volatile oils, 45% for alkaloids, 25% for glycosides and other hydrophilic compounds.

Note: Precautions, Contraindications, Kinetics, Mechanism Of Toxicity, Other

The contraindication and precaution categories contain information aimed at preventing misuse of the herbs. The means by which the botanical substances are absorbed, metabolized, and excreted are pertinent to effective therapy, evaluation of toxicity, and appropriate treatment of overdose. Information on kinetics of toxic components is therefore included in this section, also. As is the case with toxic constituents, the mechanism of toxicity may or may not be associated with the mechanism of therapeutic activity. The toxic effects may depend on other constituents, or represent an exaggerated action due to excessive exposure to the therapeutic substance. The mechanistic description is limited to the specific influences of only the most toxic substances in the plant. Other information regarding the plant part normally used medicinally, the inclusion of the toxic effects of an isolated constituent under the "Toxicity" heading, and other points of emphasis to place the information in context are also included under this heading.

Toxicity Signs/Symptoms: Internal, External, Acute, Chronic, Lab, ECG

An aspect to consider in all toxic cases is the patient's individual sensitivity to a substance and their ability to excrete it following internal exposure. Allergic sensitivities are not strictly considered as toxicities and will not be described in this section, aside from contact dermatitis from external exposure which often includes both chemical and allergic components. Toxicity signs and symptoms are listed, when possible, in the order of their appearance and growing severity. Also, effects from chronic use are differentiated from acute toxicity. If toxic constituents differ with different plant parts, the different parts will have their toxicities described separately. Since symptoms of toxicity are caused by particular toxic components, the effects of the extracted, isolated or synthesized toxic constituents are not differentiated from that of the whole plant in certain noted instances when the activity of that component is predominant. When the toxicity of an isolated constituent is included under this heading this is indicated under "Notes." Pertinent laboratory tests or electrocardiogram (ECG) changes are noted to aid monitoring.

Treatment: First Aid, Medical and Other

The best approach in any poisoning always includes immediately contacting the local poison control center for specific information regarding management of the case. The victim should be transported to a treatment facility (hospital emergency room, urgent care center, or medical clinic) if directed to do so by the poison control center or if no phone is available to call for medical advice. If neither of these measures are possible, general first aid measures, as described in numbers 1, 2, 4, 7-9 later in this section, may be followed. Under the "Treatment" heading, specific emergency first aid measures are described that do not require prescription medication. Following the first aid measures under the "Treatment" heading, specific medical intervention is described which requires assessment and treatment by a licensed doctor.

When treating toxicity medically, the degree of severity must be assessed before performing any heroic intervention. Many of the antidotal substances are potentially toxic themselves and require judicious application and then, only when vitally necessary. In counteracting toxic effects, doses may be used which normally would be prohibitive. Specific treatment should be given if the ingested plant substance is known. General medical measures are describe below in numbers 1, 3, 5, 6 and 9-15. Medical intervention needs to be accomplished by an appropriate licensed health care practitioner or emergency medical technician.

Other treatments of toxicity for certain herbs include those available to most naturopathic physicians from their own therapeutic armamentaria. The allopathic treatment of choice in these cases may differ, especially in regard to the use of substances not included in the naturopathic pharmacopeia. Homeopathic treatment may be especially useful, but it should not be the only means of treatment for acutely toxic patients. The first step is always the removal or chemical neutralization of the toxic substance. It is important for naturopaths to be aware of specific chemical antidotes that they are not permitted to use, so that they can act properly in cases where they are unable to manage toxicities by means within the scope of their legal practice. Therefore, the treatment of toxicities according to the standard medical protocol is first briefly outlined to facilitate appropriate assessment, management, or referral.

Ordinarily, the following general approach in treating toxicities should be pursued.

1. The first concern is the maintenance of respiration and circulation. Cardiopulmonary resusitation should be administered when indicated. Establish an artificial airway if necessary. A normal tidal volume of 10-15 cc/kg is desired.

2. Of essential importance is to quickly minimize absorption of the toxic substance. This is initially attempted by emptying the stomach, if emesis (vomiting) can be accomplished within an hour of ingestion of the poison. Spontaneous vomiting often fulfills this need. Otherwise, syrup of ipecac can be employed (15cc = 1/2 oz. = 1 tablespoon for children; 30cc for adults), followed with a large amount of water (8 oz. for children; 16 oz. for adults). Get the victim to walk and stimulate the back of his or her throat. If necessary, repeat in 20-30 minutes. Mustard powder (1/2 - 1 Tbs.) or lobelia tincture (1/2 - 1 tsp.) in one cup of warm water are not as reliable and have toxic properties of their own, but they may be adequate if no ipecac is available. One tablespoon of salt in a glass of warm water has less potential toxicity than ipecac, mustard powder or lobelia but is an unreliable emetic. Emesis is contraindicated in coma, convulsions, or loss of gag reflex, because of the possibility of asphyxia or aspirational pneumonitis. Vomiting petroleum distillates or essential oils may also lead to pneumonitis. Vomiting is further contraindicated following the ingestion of corrosive chemical agents, since more severe damage to the esophagus, throat and mouth can result with re-exposure to the corrosive material. (See "Contraindicated" under Notes section for *Cephalis ipecachuana* for additional conditions for which ipecac and other emetics should not be used.)

3. When emesis is contraindicated, as in the consumption of petroleum distillates or corrosives, endotracheal intubation is done prior to gastric lavage. Lavage with copious normal saline in a 36-50 French orogastric hose; use the head-down, left-side position with suction, and save the aspirate.

4. After emptying the stomach, further absorption may be prevented by administering activated charcoal at 5-10 times the ingested dose, or from 30-50 grams, in a water slurry. Repeat, if necessary. This not only absorbs many alkaloidal substances, but also blackens the stool, so that passage of the toxic substances from the body may be noted.

5. If diarrhea is not a presenting symptom, the use of a cathartic to eliminate the toxins from the bowel should be considered. Here, saline cathartics are to be used rather than irritating anthroquinone-containing herbal laxatives, since the bowel mucosa may already be chemically irritated. Oral sodium or magnesium sulfate is advised (250 mg/kg for children; 20-30 grams/dose up to 100 grams total for adults of Epsom salts). Magnesium cathartics are contraindicated in renal failure. Catharsis is contraindicated following ingestion of corrosive material to avoid causing more extensive damage to the intestinal tract.

6. Alkaloidal toxins can be rendered nonabsorbable by precipitation. Tannins from herbs or common store tea will precipitate most alkaloidal toxins. Such teas should be administered with sodium bicarbonate to maintain the precipitate; the stomach should then be emptied. Potassium permanganate (15-50 grains in a pint of water) may be used as a precipitating agent with gastric lavage if there is no organic matter present in the stomach, and it must not be left in the stomach. Tincture of iodine or Lugol's solution may also be used to precipitate alkaloids, but it redissolves in the alkalinity of the intestines, and so should be removed speedily (for example, with a purgative).

These agents are best employed together with gastric lavage to ensure their complete removal.

7. For dermal exposure to toxins, the patient should be removed from the source. Clothing and all exposed areas should be washed twice with soap and water. Scratching should be prevented and lenitives applied for pain or itching. These measures help to prevent the spread of the toxin and the resultant dermatitis. Absorption of poisonous substances through the skin may lead to systemic toxicities requiring further treatment.

8. In eye exposure, irrigate copiously with water for 15 minutes. If pain persists, refer for ophthalmic exam.

9. Allergic sensitivities may include an entire plant family for a sensitive individual (for example, Asteraceae). Symptomatic treatment of the resultant rash, itching, or congestion may be used until a desensitization program can be established.

10. For gastroenteritis with nausea, vomiting, or diarrhea, monitor fluid and electrolytes and replace as necessary. Obtain pertinent lab tests for baseline function studies. In the recovery phase, demulcents may be used, such as slippery elm mucilage, acacia, flaxseed tea, oatmeal gruel, and others. If pain and irritation persist, opiates or anticholinergics may be employed cautiously.

11. Hypotension is best treated with fluids; a vasopressor is used only when absolutely necessary.

12. In CNS depression, maintain breathing with a respirator and treat for cerebral edema with hypertonic urea (1 gram/kg) or 20% mannitol (5-10 ml/kg) given over a thirty minute period.

13. Convulsions may be treated rectally with an antispasmotic tincture if IV diazepam (0.1 - 0.3 mg/kg in children; up to 10 mg in adults) is unavailable.

14. In depressive poisoning, the following may be considered for their stimulative properties: coffee as needed; aromatic spirit of ammonia (1 tsp every 10-15 minutes). Atropine sulphate (1/100 grain subcutaneously) is suitable for cardiac and respiratory depression.

15. If the ingested toxins are known to be eliminated in the urine, forcing fluids orally and rectally may be considered. To prevent reabsorption, try to produce alkaline urine for acidic toxins and acidic urine for alkaline toxins.

References

Although much of the information obtained on the adverse effects of plant products used clinically was recovered from the Eclectic medical texts by Felter (1922) and Ellingwood (1919), more recent scientific information on toxicology has been included to update these works. The only other older texts used are *A Modern Herbal*, a standard herbalist reference originally published in 1931, and *Naturae Medicina and Naturopathic Dispensatory* (1953), the text which served as a basic naturopathic materia medica since its publication.

Although much of the information provided is from recently published works, these sources should not be divorced from knowledge gleaned over the past several hundred years. Modern references mainly provide a scientifically-established explanation of the long-established medicinal action of herbs. All the information presented on a given plant is from the references listed for that plant, with the exception of the chemical classifications of alkaloids, glycosides, and volatile oils. These chemical categories, as listed in the index of toxic constituents, are all taken from the book *Pharmacognosy*, 7th ed., by Tyler, Brady & Robbers (1976), which may or may not otherwise be listed as a reference on that herb's toxicity.

The definitive American text on poisonous plants, *Poisonous Plants of the United States and Canada* by John M. Kingsbury (1964), is not listed as a reference for this book, since the information from Dr. Kingsbury's book was used as a basis for information on plants in the Poisindex data base. This authority is therefore represented here as well.

Primary references for the appendices specifically address the issues raised there, i.e., the toxicity of essential oils and herbs contraindicated in pregnancy. For the former, *Essential Oil Safety* is the text which should be referred to for those who want comprehensive information on this topic. For pregnancy reliance was made on an extensive literature search documenting folk medicine and scientific findings associated with uterine stimulant effects of plants published in the *Journal of Pharmaceutical Sciences* in 1975. Other texts and articles have been added to complement these major references.

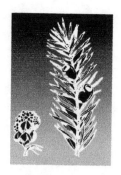

THE
TOXICOLOGY

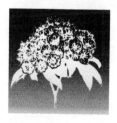

OF
BOTANICAL
MEDICINES

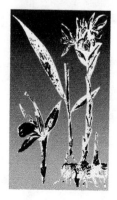

THE TOXICOLOGY OF BOTANICAL MEDICINES

Aconitum napellus L.; *Aconitum* spp.   Ranunculaceae

Common Names:

Monkshood, wolfsbane, friar's cap, mousebane; aconite

Parts Containing Toxins:

Whole herb, especially roots and seeds.

Toxic Constituents – Aconitine, mesaconitine, hypaconitine, 3-acetylacoitine, lappaconitine, (diterpenoid-ester alkaloids), benzaconine, benzoylaconine.

Doses:

Therapeutic – Fluid extract 1 drop (0.06 ml); tincture 1-8 drops (0.06-0.49 ml); aconitine crystals 0.13 mg). Processed Chinese roots 1.5-3.0 gm.

Toxic – Tincture > 10 drops (0.62 ml); decoction of 6 gm cured rootstock. Aconitine 0.2 mg.

Lethal – Powder 1 gram, 5 ml of tincture, or 2 mg of aconitine.

Note:

Kinetics – Aconitine is absorbed through mucous membranes and the skin. Symptoms develop as quickly as 3 minutes, in an average of 30 minutes, and always within 2 hours.

Mechanism of Toxicity – The aconitines, except for lappaconitine, activate the sodium and calcium channels, stimulating and then depressing the myocardium, smooth muscles, skeletal muscles, central nervous system, and peripheral nerves. In the heart the overall activity prolongs repolarization in the myocytes and causes after depolarizations and triggered automaticity leading to ventricular tachyarrhythmias and other arrhythmias. Lappaconitine acts as an antagonist, blocking the sodium and calcium channels and having antiarrhythmia and bradycardia effects. Nociceptive effects are due to all of these alkaloids. Muscarinic activation also accounts for subsequent bradyarrhythmias and hypotension.

Other – The mind remains clear in the poisoning process.

The toxicity of the plant parts follows the order of their alkaloid content: roots > flowers > leaves > stems.

The toxicity of dried roots from Asian *Aconitum* species such as the Chinese *Aconitum carmichaeli*, *Aconitum kusnezoffii*, and *Aconitum brachypodium* is typically reduced by proper processing involving soaking or boiling prior to medicinal use. Inadequate root decoction time during preparation can prevent necessary hydrolysis of the aconitines to the less toxic aconines.

Monkshood is among the most poisonous of all plants known to humans.

Toxicity Signs/Symptoms:

Tingling or burning of the tongue followed by numbness of the mouth, throat, and hands; nausea and vomiting with epigastric pain, a sensation of ants crawling over the body; labored breathing with weak pulse; giddiness, staggering, dizziness, restlessness, loss of speech control, hypersalivation, diarrhea; intense headache, pinpoint pupils, blurred vision; hypotension; irregular heartbeat and breathing, chest pain, shallow respirations, skin cold and clammy; ventricular tachycardia or fibrillation in about 2 hours (1-6 hours); sweating and hypothermia; patient is cold and cannot stand; the face is pale, the eyes sunken; slow and weak pulse, extreme anxiety; muscular weakness, tetraplegia; loss of consciousness, convulsions and death due to respiratory failure or cardiac arrest within hours even in small doses.

Lab – EEG may show changes associated with myocardial infanct.

Treatment:

First Aid – CPR; activated charcoal orally, then emesis; recumbent posture with head lower than feet; keep patient warm and quiet.

Medical – O_2 and/or mechanical ventilation as needed; gastric lavage; magnesium and calcium infusions; digitalization for cardiac depression; amiodarone or flecainide for ventricular tachycardia; atropine to prevent slowing of heart; antiarrhythmic drugs such as lidocaine or bretylium, or cardiopulmonary bypass as last resort for refractory ventricular fibrillation.

Other – Tannic acid with emetic and cathartic; stimulants such as coffee or nux vomica as needed; if not retained, diluted brandy injected rectally. Friction rub.

References:

1, 3, 5, 6, 7, 8, 9, 10, 14, 101, 103, 104, 107, 116, 117, 118, 119, 164, 165

Acorus calamus L.   Acaceae

Common Names:

Calamus, sweet flag, grass myrtle, myrtle flag, sweet grass, sweet myrtle, sweet rush, sweet root, sweet cane, myrtle sedge

Parts Containing Toxins:

Rhizome

Toxic Constituents – Oil with alpha- and beta-asarone (volatile ethers).

Doses:

Therapeutic – Tincture 1.85-3.7 ml.

Toxic – Tincture (1:2) LD_{50} 5 ml/kg IP in mice. Oil chronic dietary levels of 500-5,000 ppm are carcinogenic in animals.

Note:

Precautions – Avoid long-term use.

Contraindications – In pregnancy due to emmenagogue and potential abortifacient effects of the Asian and European varieties. (Commercial sources may not differentiate these in labelling.) The oil should not be used internally or externally in therapy.

Mechanism of Toxicity – The ethanolic extract acts as a mild CNS depressant. Alpha-asarone accounts for some, but not all, of its neurodepressive activity. Beta-asarone is reportedly hallucinogenic. The beta-asarone produces mutagenic effects and is procarcinogenic in lab studies in high doses.

Other – Reference 14 lists this plant as nontoxic. Reference 100 distinguishes the nontoxic American variety (*americanus*) whose volatile oil does not contain beta-asarone from the oils of the toxic Asian (*angustatus*) and European (*calamus*) varieties which contain 80-96% and less than 10%, respectively.

Toxicity Signs/Symptoms:

Acute [In animals] – Drowsiness, tremors, convulsions.

Chronic –Growth depression, ascites; kidney, heart and liver changes, possibly intestinal malignancies.

Treatment:

(See Treatment section under Explanation of Format.)

References:

2, 5, 14, 25, 100, 104, 105, 107, 120

Actea alba Big.;
Actea spicata L.   Ranunculaceae

Common Names:

White cohosh, white baneberry, necklace weed, white beads; baneberry, bugbane, toadroot, herb Christopher

Parts Containing Toxins:

Whole herb, especially root and berries, stalk and sap.

Toxic Constituents – Protoanemonin (lactone).

Doses:

Therapeutic – Rhizome powder 65-1296 mg; tincture 1-30 drops (0.06-1.85 ml).

Toxic – A few berries.

Note:

Mechanism of Toxicity – The plant is a mucous membrane irritation.

Other – Symptoms appear within 30 minutes and last one hour. Patient returns to normal in three hours.

Toxicity Signs/Symptoms:

External – Skin rashes and eye irritation.

Internal – Severe gastritis, bloody diarrhea, headache, vomiting, dysuria, hematuria, circulatory failure, incoherence, visual hallucination, stomach cramps, dizziness, tachycardia.

Treatment:

First Aid – Emesis; activated charcoal. For contact dermatitis remove from source, wash clothing and exposed area twice with soap and water, and prevent scratching.

Medical – Gastric lavage; cathartic; maintain fluid and electrolyte balance.

References:

3, 5, 6, 8, 12, 14, 103

Adonis vernalis L.   **Ranunculaceae**

Common Names:

Pheasant's eye, false hellebore , sweet vernal

Parts Containing Toxins:

Aerial herb.

Toxic Constituents – Adonitoxin, adonidin, cymarin, K-strophanthin (steroid glycosides) and about two dozen other cardenolides.

Doses:

Therapeutic – Powder 0.5-1.0 gm; fluid extract 1-2 drops (0.06-0.12 ml); Adonidin 6.5-21.6 mg.

Note:

> **Contraindications** – Potassium deficiency or digitalis glycoside therapy.

> **Kinetics** – Between 15-37% of the cardioactive glycosides are absorbed. Their half-lives are from 13-23 hours, and the duration of action is about 2.8 days. They are mainly excreted through the kidneys.

> **Mechanism of Toxicity** – Besides acting on the heart like digitaloids, it also produces gastrointestinal irritation.

> **Other** –Enhanced toxicity with quinidine, calcium, diuretics, laxatives, and chronic glucocorticoid therapy.

Toxicity Signs/Symptoms:

> Vomiting, diarrhea, cardiac arrhythmias or heart paralysis.

Treatment:

> **First Aid** – Emesis or gastric lavage; activated charcoal; cathartic.

> **Medical** – Atropine to restore atrial activity and raise heart rate at dosage 0.6 mg IV for adults, 0.05 mg/kg/dose IV in children. Phenytoin; transvenous electrical pacer; hyperkalemia should be monitored and treated with Kayeralate (R) or glucose and insulin.

References:

> 3, 6, 7, 12, 14, 93, 103, 106, 107

Aesculus hippocastanum L.   **Hippocastanaceae**

Common Names:

> Horse chestnut, buckeye, Spanish chestnut

Parts Containing Toxins:

> Bark, leaves, and the nonmedicinal flowers, pericarp of the green fruit, and twigs.

> **Toxic Constituents** – Esculin (hydroxycoumarin lactone glycoside) in leaves, bark, buds, and pericarp of fruit.

Doses:

> **Therapeutic** – Seed extract 300 mg (50 mg escin); esculin 4 mg once daily.

> **Toxic** – A few fruit can cause severe symptoms.

> **Lethal** – In children, a few fruit may cause death.

Note:

> **Mechanism of Toxicity** – Neural stimulation and also increased antithrombin activity by the hydroxycoumarin esculin leads to increased bleeding time. Produces mucous membrane irritation.

> **Other** – Roasting seems to destroy the toxins.

> The seed is the part normally used in medicine. Some use of the bark also occurs.

Toxicity Signs/Symptoms:

> Nausea, vomiting, inflamed membranes, diarrhea, weakness, dizziness, incoordination, paralysis, increased temperature, strabismus, vertigo, amblyopia, torticollis, opisthotonus, mental stupor, coma; also depression, nervous twitching, hemolysis, mydriasis, fever; possibly elation; death due to respiratory paralysis.

Treatment:

> **First Aid** – Establish adequate respiration, emesis, charcoal. For contact dermatitis wash clothing and exposed area twice with soap and water and avoid scratching.

> **Medical** – Gastric lavage, cathartic; maintain fluid and electrolyte balance.

References:

> 1, 3, 5, 7, 9, 10, 12, 14, 88, 104

Aletris farinosa L.   Liliaceae

Common Names:

Blazing star, stargrass, true unicorn, starwort

Parts Containing Toxins:

Root.

Toxic Constituents – Probably volatile oil and resin.

Doses:

Therapeutic – Dried root 0.3-0.6 grams; tincture 15-40 drops (0.93-2.47 ml).

Note:

Contraindications – In pregnancy since uterine stimulant activity has been shown in animals.

Toxicity Signs/Symptoms:

Narcotic, emetic and cathartic

Treatment:

(See Treatment section under Explanation of Format.)

References:

5, 25

Aloe ferox Mill.;
Aloe vera (L.) N.L. Burm.
(= *Aloe barbadensis* Mill.)   Liliaceae

Common Names:

Aloes, Cape aloe; Barbadoes aloe, Curacao aloe, hepatic aloes

Parts Containing Toxins:

Dried latex from leaves.

Toxic Constituents – Aloin A and B and aloinoside A and B (anthraquinone glycosides) (not in *A. vera* gel) and aloeresin A. *A. vera* also contains 7-hydroxyaloins.

Doses:

Therapeutic – Powder 16.2 mg; tincture 15-60 drops (0.93-3.7 ml).

Note:

Precaution – Do not use in excess of 8-10 days. Loss of potassium can enhance cardiac glycoside effects.

Contraindications – In pregnancy and in menstruation, especially menorrhagia and metrorrhagia, and actively inflamed hemorrhoids. Also in intestinal obstruction, abdominal pain of unknown origin, any intestinal inflammation, in kidney dysfunction, and in children under twelve.

Mechanism of Toxicity – Anthraquinone glycosides act as intestinal irritants and stimulate active intestinal chloride secretion. The resultant laxative effect potentiates its action as an emmenagogue and potential abortifacient.

Other – The latex from the similar species *Aloe perryi* has equivalent effects and contraindications. The juice, or gel, from the leaves is commonly used topically for damage to the skin.

Toxicity Signs/Symptoms:

Diarrhea with griping; rectal discomfort; possibly nausea and vomiting; nephritis.

Treatment:

First Aid – Emesis; charcoal.

Medical – Gastric lavage if no emesis.

Other – Demulcents.

References:

3, 5, 9, 10, 11, 14, 25, 32, 100, 101, 106, 107

Amanita muscaria Pers.   **Polyporaceae**

Common Names:

Fly agaric, fly amanita

Parts Containing Toxins:

Whole fungus.

Toxic Constituents – Ibotenic acid and muscimol (isoxazole derivatives), muscazone (oxazole derivative), small amounts of muscarine (alkaloid); stizololic acid, tricholomic acid.

Doses:

Therapeutic – Tincture 1/30 drop (0.2 mcl).

Toxic – 2-4 mushrooms (> 10 gm fresh).

Lethal – 20 mushrooms (> 100 gm fresh).

Note:

Mechanism of Toxicity – Muscarine stimulates postganglionic cholinergic neuroeffector junctions.

The isoxazole constituents are psychoactive.

Other – Higher concentrations of muscarine are contained in *Inocybe* spp. and *Clitocybe* spp. (3% when dried) without the other toxins, giving a more purely cholinergic effect. Symptoms appear 10-15 hours after ingestion. The following toxicity symptoms are given for the isolated toxic constituents.

Toxicity Signs/Symptoms:

Mushrooms – Vomiting, abdominal pain, dizziness, muscle cramps, twitching, poor coordination; confusion, mental stimulation, illusions, manic attacks, then profound sleep; depression, unconsciousness, asphyxiation, death.

Isoxazoles – Irritability, restlessness, ataxia, hallucination, delirium.

Muscarine – Malaise, increased salivation, perspiration and lacrimation; excessive thirst, nausea, vomiting, diarrhea; abdominal and extremity cramping, cerebral excitement; headache, anuria, muscular weakness, miosis, tetanic peristalsis, paralysis, slow pulse, rapid breathing, fall in blood pressure, depression, coma, heart collapses in diastole (respiratory failure also possible); shock. The autopsy shows fatty degeneration of heart, liver and kidneys. If not lethal, hemolysis eventually leads to jaundice with interstitial nephritis and uremia.

Treatment:

>   **First Aid** – Emesis; activated charcoal; CPR.

>   **Medical** – Gastric lavage. Do not automatically use atropine as antagonist; only use if indicated by cholinergic effects. Hypertonic glucose intravenously; sedation when required initially, followed by stimulants if necessary.

>   **Other** – Colonic irrigation; treatment is variable, according to symptoms. Supportive care for respiration, circulation, and pulmonary edema if indicated.

References:

>   3, 6, 7, 9, 13, 14, 107

Ammi visnaga (L.) Lam.   Apiaceae

Common Names:

>   Khella, bishop's weed

Parts Containing Toxins:

>   Fruit (seeds).

>   **Toxic Constituents** – 1.1% Khellin, 0.7% visnagin (furochromones); visnadin, samidin (pyranocoumarins).

Doses:

>   **Therapeutic** – Khellin 50-100 mg.

>   **Toxic** – Khellin 100 mg.

>   **Lethal** – Khellin LD_{50} 0.08 gm/kg orally in rats.

Note:

>   **Precautions** – Avoid excessive exposure to ultraviolet light after use.

>   **Contraindications** – In pregnancy due to its emmenagogue effect and the uterine stimulant action of the component khellin.

>   **Mechanism of Toxicity** – The furochromones are potent vasodilators. The pyranocoumarins may be phototoxic and are cAMP-phosphodiesterase inhibitors.

Other – The volatile oil contains 1% khellin.

Toxicity Signs/Symptoms:

Nausea, loss of appetite, headache, dizziness, sleep disorders.

Lab – Elevated liver enzymes.

Treatment:

(See Treatment section under Explanation of Format.)

References:

25, 39, 40, 86, 87, 105, 107, 213, 214

Anamirta cocculus (L.) **Wight et Arnott**
(=*Anamirta panniculata* Col.)
Menispermaceae

Common Names:

Fishberries, Indian berries, cocculus, levant nut

Parts Containing Toxins:

Fruit with seeds.

Toxic Constituents – 1.5% Picrotoxin (sesquiterpene glycoside).

Doses:

Therapeutic – Fruit 1-5 mg daily; picrotoxin 0.43-1.0 mg.

Toxic – Picrotoxin 20 mg; a few berries.

Lethal – 2-3 berries.

Note:

Precaution – Do not use on abraded or open surfaces nor in large quantities.

Mechanism of Toxicity – A powerful stimulant affecting all portions of the CNS by blocking inhibitory synapses, being antagonistic to GABA. Seems to most affect medullary centers controlling respiration and circulation.

Other – Used as a fish poison in Asia.

Toxicity Signs/Symptoms:

Nausea, GI irritation, headache, dizziness, twitching muscles, trembling; salivation, vomiting, rapid breathing, slow pulse, cardiac palpitation, hypertension; alternate clonic and tonic convulsions with tonic flexion preceding tonic extension, depression insensibility, sleepiness, coma, death through respiratory paralysis or heart failure sometimes days after ingestion.

Treatment:

First Aid – Emesis, activated charcoal.

Medical – Gastric lavage if no emesis; purge with sodium sulphate; diuretics; administer anticonvulsives and cardiac stimulants such as diazepam and digitalis, respectively. Avoid phenothiazines and analeptics.

Other – In case of fever wrap in ice packs, administer glucose and oxygen.

References:

3, 7, 9, 13, 107

Apocynum androsaemifolium L.,
Apocynum cannabinum L.   Apocynaceae

Common Names:

Dogbane, catchfly, Indian hemp, Canadian hemp, bitter root, fly trap

Parts Containing Toxins:

Roots, entire plant.

Toxic Constituents – Apocynin (saponin); cymarin and K-strophanthin, plus apocannosides in *A. cannabinum* (steroid glycosides).

Doses:

Therapeutic – Fluid extract 10-30 drops (0.62-1.85 ml).

Lethal – Infusion 0.86 ml/kg (IV in cats) of *A. androsaemifolium*

Note:

Mechanism of Toxicity – Besides acting on the heart like *Digitalis* spp., it also produces gastrointestinal irritation more than other cardioactive drugs.

Other – A dose of 0.1 gram of the root possesses a potency of 2 USP digitalis units. *A. cannabinum* extract fraction produced faster and greater inotropic effect than digitalin (*in vitro*)

One toxicity report confused this plant with *Nerium oleander*.

Toxicity Signs/Symptoms:

Nausea, vomiting and diarrhea, diaphoresis; cardiac arrhythmias and depressed pulse rate; increased blood pressure; possible death.

Treatment:

First Aid – Emesis or gastric lavage; activated charcoal.

Medical – Cathartic; atropine 0.6 mg IV adults, 0.05 mg/kg/dose IV children; phenytoin; transvenous electrical pacemaker if necessary; monitor for hyperkalemia and treat with Kayeralate (R) or glucose and insulin.

References:

3, 5, 9, 10, 12, 14, 75, 76, 77, 78, 107

Areca catechu L.   **Arecaceae**

Common Names:

Betel nut, areca nut , pinang

Parts Containing Toxins: Seed.

Toxic Constituents – Arecoline, arecain (pyridine alkaloids).

Doses:

Toxic – Seed 8-10 gm; fluid extract 3.7 ml; arecoline hydrobromide 4.3-6.5 mg.

Note:

Contraindications – In pregnancy due to the teratogenic and fetotoxic effects in mice.

Mechanism of Toxicity – The seed causes parasympathomimetic action with cortical arousal. Arecoline is converted to the CNS stimulant arecaidine by chewing. Chewing also releases carcinogenic nitrosamines.

Other – Carcinogenesis has been shown to occur in mice and rats with both cured and uncured seed extracts with continual exposure.

Toxicity Signs/Symptoms:

Acute – Vomiting, diarrhea, difficult breathing; salivation, sweating, tremors, slow heart rate, impaired vision, miosis, mydriasis, intestinal cramps, convulsions; paralysis, coma, death.

Chronic – Malignant tumors in mouth from chewing.

Treatment:

First Aid – Emesis; activated charcoal.

Medical – Gastric lavage if no emesis; atropine (2 mg subcut), repeat if necessary; counteract pulmonary edema to avoid respiratory embarrassment; observe vital signs for supportive care of circulatory insufficiency; IV diazepam for seizures.

References:

1, 13, 14, 21, 37, 103, 107

Aristolochia serpentaria L.;
Aristolochia spp.   **Aristolochiaceae**

Common Names:

Virginia snakeroot, serpentaria, pelican flower, red river snakeroot, snakeweed, thick birthwort, sangree root, Texas snakeroot; birthwort, Chinese aristolochia

Parts Containing Toxins:

Dried rhizomes and roots.

Toxic Constituents – Aristolochin, aristolochic acid.

Doses:

Therapeutic – Powder 65-1944 mg; tincture 5-25 drops (0.62-1.54 ml).

Toxic – Powder from *A. fanchi* 100-200 mg three times daily for 5 months.

Note:

Contraindications – In active fever or severe inflammation and in pregnancy. In additon to being highly toxic, *Aristolochia clematis* (birthwort) has oxytocic and abortifacient effects.

Mechanism of Toxicity – Bitter components can paralyze the respiration. Aristolochic acid is toxic to the kidneys and is carcinogenic and mutagenic in animals and human cells.

Other – Case reports of toxicity from consuming *Aristolochia pistolochia* and *Aristolochia fanchi* confirm the nephrotoxicity. Other medicinal species including *Aristolochia clematitis, Aristolochia contorta, Aristolochia debilis,* and *Asarum canadense* also contain the toxic aristolochic acid.

Toxicity Signs/Symptoms:

Acute – Gastric irritation, headache, vertigo, nausea, vomiting; diarrhea with griping pain and tenesmus; drowsiness, but with disturbed sleep.

Chronic – Progressive renal failure.

Lab – Elevated serum creatinine and renal biopsy findings of interstitial sclerosis, tubular atrophy, and thickening of Bowmman's capsule and interlobular arteriole walls with chronic consumption.

Treatment:

(See Treatment section under Explanation of Format.)

References:

3, 5, 9, 100, 104, 107, 121, 122, 123, 166

Arnica montana L.   Asteraceae

Common Names:

Leopard's bane, wolfsbane, mountain tobacco

Parts Containing Toxins:

Flowers and roots.

Toxic Constituents - Arnicine, formic acid; thymohydroquinone (volatile oil); arnifolin, helenalin, helenalin acetate (sesquiterpene lactones).

Doses:

Therapeutic – Flower tincture 1-10 drops (0.06-0.62 ml).

Lethal – Tincture 2 oz (59.2 ml).

Note:

Precaution – Do not use over any break in the skin, nor topically as an undiluted tincture; those with gout or sensitive skin are the most affected by topical use.

Contraindications – In pregnancy since it has been shown to be a uterine stimulant. Also, in those who are allergic to sesquiterpene lactones in the Asteracea family.

Mechanism of Toxicity – Arnica acts as an irritant and blocks nerve function, especially the vagus, in large doses. Sesquiterpene lactones can cause contact dermatitis which can sensitive individuals to similar compounds in related Asteracea plants.

Other – In Europe the extract is now only approved for topical, not internal, use.

The species *Arnica longifolia* has also been shown to induce dermatitis due to its sesquiterpene lactone content.

Toxicity Signs/Symptoms:

Internal – Gastric burning, nausea, vomiting, diarrhea; restlessness, headache, decreased temperature, dyspnea, drowsiness, muscular weakness, decrease in pulse rate, cardiovascular collapse; convulsions, coma, death.

External – Dermal irritation deepening into an erysipelatous or acute eczematous inflammation, with pustules and blisters.

Treatment:

First Aid – Emesis, activated charcoal.

Medical – Gastric lavage; if early, do lavage with a liter of potassium permanganate diluted 1:10,000 to inactivate the alkaloids in the stomach; cathartic; observe four hours;

IV diazepam for seizures; dopamine or phenylephrine for hypotension.

References:

1, 3, 5, 6, 9, 10, 14, 25, 100, 101, 106, 107, 124, 125

Artemisia absinthium L.   Asteraceae

Common Names:

Wormwood, absinthe

Parts Containing Toxins:

Flowering tops and leaves.

Toxic Constituents – Oil with absinthol, thujone, and d-isothujone (volatile ketones).

Doses:

Therapeutic – Powder 970-1300 mg; tincture 10-30 drops (0.6-1.8 ml); oil 1-5 drops (0.05-0.25 ml).

Toxic – Oil 10 ml.

Lethal – Oil LD_{50} 0.96 gm/kg in animals; thujone LD_{50} 0.21 mg/kg orally in animals.

Note:

Contraindications – In pregnancy since it is an emmenagogue in humans and uterine stimulant in animals. The oil should not be used internally or externally in therapy.

Mechanism of Toxicity – Thujone is neurotoxic and can cause CNS depression.

Other – As contained in the beverages Absinthe and Vermouth, it may be habit forming. In Germany the essential oil is not approved for oral use. The volatile oils of related species such as *Artemisia herba-alba, Artemisia abrotanum,* and *Artemisia arborescens* are quite toxic due to their thujone content, and so also have the same contraindication as *A. absinthium.*

Toxicity Signs/Symptoms:

Acute – Vomiting, GI cramps, headache, trembling, dizziness, then stupor, followed by clonic convulsions, death.

Chronic – Disturbed rest; disagreeable dreams; morning nausea and vomiting, vertigo; epileptoid attacks; physical and mental force impaired; impotence or premature menopause; hyperesthesia of the hypogastrium. Liver damage.

External – Dermatitis.

Treatment:

First Aid – [Acute] Emesis; activated charcoal.

Medical – [Acute] Gastric lavage; cathartic; maintain fluid and electrolyte balance; avoid use of drugs.

References:

3, 5, 6, 9, 14, 25, 74, 100, 101, 105, 106, 107

Artemisia cina O.C. Berg et C.F. Schmidt;
Artemisia maritima L.;
Artemisia pauciflora Web.   **Asteraceae**

Common Names:

Levant wormseed; sea wormwood; santonica

Parts Containing Toxins:

Unopened flowerheads, whole plant.

Toxic Constituents – Santonin, artemisin (sesquiterpene lactones 1-7%).

Doses:

Therapeutic – Powder 1-2 gm; santonin crystals 6.5-260 mg.

Toxic – Santonin 60 mg in children, 200 mg in adult.

Lethal – Flowers 10 gm; santonin 15 mg/kg body weight, as little as 325 mg in normal child, 130 mg in feeble child. Santonin LD_{50} 900 mg/kg orally, 180 mg/kg IV, and 130 mg/kg IP in mice.

Note:

Precaution – Excessive alkalinity in the intestines increases its absorption and toxicity.

Kinetics – Most santonin is eliminated unchanged in the feces. What is absorbed is oxidized and excreted in the urine. Elimination is slow, so santonin can acts as a cumulative poison when taken in therapeutic doses for too long of a time. Santonin crosses the placenta and is also secreted in mothers' milk. To reduce absorption santonin should be given a few hours after meals with fats excluded from the diet for 12 hours prior.

Mechanism of Toxicity – It acts as a motor stimulant on the CNS and may cause hypermia of the brain. Anticholinesterase activity has been reported. Retinal violet receptors are first stimulated, then depressed. Irritation and inflammation of the mucosa occur locally.

Other – Santonin stains tissues yellow, including the nails.

Santonin is most effective when combined with a saline laxative, but not castor oil which increases its absorption. The following refers to the effects of santonin derived from *Artemisia* spp.

Toxicity Signs/Symptoms:

Internal – Abdominal cramps; nausea and vomiting; visual disorders including xanthopsia or chromatopsia commonly occur early; coldness and pallor; headaches; profuse sweating, hearing difficulties, vertigo; generalized asthenia, apathy; kidney irritation, painful urination, anuria; diarrhea; profuse sweating; flushed face, salivation and foaming at the mouth; swollen spleen, reduced body temperature; disturbed smell and taste;

mydriasis, tears; acid urine color from bright yellow to orange or saffron; alkaline urine is reddish-purple; dilated pupils; decreased blood pressure; bradycardia; twitching eyes and head; clenching of teeth; hallucinations, stupefaction, dizziness, delirium, giddiness; epileptiform convulsions; tetany or cramps; paralysis of the legs, unconsciousness and death by respiratory paralysis or cardiac failure. If nonfatal, aphasia or temporary blindness may result.

Lab – Albunimuria, hematuria.

External - Dermatitis can occur when handling fresh plant.

Treatment:

First Aid – CPR; charcoal. For contact dermatitis wash twice with soap and water.

Medical – Gastric lavage, saline catharsis and support against convulsions and collapse; maintain fluid and electrolytes.

Other – Strong coffee and spirit of ammonia.

References:

3, 7, 9, 10, 14, 102, 103, 107

Asclepias tuberosa L.   **Asclepiadaceae**

Common Names:

Pleurisy root, butterfly weed, Canada root, flux root, orange swallow-wort, tuber root, white root, wind root

Parts Containing Toxins:

Whole herb (including root), stems and leaves.

Toxic Constituents – Galitoxin and similar resins; glucofrugoside (cardenolide).

Doses:

Therapeutic – Root powder 1.3-1.9 gm; tincture 1/2-1 tsp (1.85-3.7 ml); fluid extract 5-30 drops (0.31-1.85 ml).

Toxic – alcoholic extract of root equivalent to 40 mg/animal (IP in rats) for ten days

Lethal – alcoholic extract of root equivalent to 32 mg/kg (IV in rabbits)

Note:

Contraindications – In pregnancy due to estrogenic effects and uterine stimulant activity in animals. The similarly-used species *Asclepias asperula* (inmortal) should also be avoided in pregnancy.

Mechanism of Toxicity – The resins are mucous membrane irritants. The cardenolides cause a slight increase in cardiac tone and slight decrease in rate and amplitude.

Other – Only the root is used medicinally.

Toxicity is reduced by drying.

Toxicity Signs/Symptoms:

Nausea and vomiting; gastrointestinal upset; diarrhea; CNS depression; muscle weakness, anorexia; staggering; death due to respiratory paralysis in one to several days.

Treatment:

First Aid – Emesis; activated charcoal.

Medical – Gastric lavage if no emesis; cathartic; maintain fluid and electrolyte balance; avoid use of drugs.

References:

3, 5, 9, 10, 14, 25, 79, 80, 81, 100

Atropa belladonna L.   Solanaceae

Common Names:

Deadly nightshade, dwale, devil's cherries, poison black cherry

Parts Containing Toxins:

Roots and leaves, berries and flowers, especially when mature.

Toxic Constituents – 0.1-0.6% Atropine produced during extraction from hyoscyamine in plant; scopolamine, also called hyoscine (tropane alkaloids, 0.3-0.7% in leaves and 0.4-0.6% in roots).

Mechanism of Toxicity – The alkaloids are competitive antagonists to acetylcholine at peripheral nerves. Scopolamine is a CNS depressant; atropine is a CNS stimulant. Actions reversed in excess.

Doses:

Therapeutic – Leaf or root powder 0.05-0.10 gm; tincture of leaves (0.03% atropine) 1-15 drops (USP 0.6-0.9 ml); extract USP 15 mg (0.2 mg atropine); scopolamine hydrobromide, 0.6 mg; atropine sulfate 0.32-1.08 mg (0.5 mg average dose).

Toxic – More than 3 berries.

Lethal – Powder 5-50 gm; 3 berries in children; atropine 10-100 mg.

Note:

Precautions – Do not use in large or continuous doses. Children are especially susceptible.

Contraindications – In glaucoma

Kinetics – Decreased GI motility caused by atropine delays absorption.

Mechanism of Toxicity – The anticholinergic alkaloids have parasympatholytic effects, especially relaxation of smooth muscles and reduced secretions and increased heart rate.

Other – The root is the most poisonous, the leaves and flowers less, and the berries the least. Even handling the plant with cuts or abrasions on the hands can cause poisoning.

The following toxicity symptoms apply to belladonna or its alkaloids.

Toxicity Signs/Symptoms:

Dry mouth, mydriasis, increased pulse rate; flushing (from face to neck to shoulders, with subsequent desquamation possible); hot and dry skin; increased respiratory rate and volume; increased temperature in children; palpitations; increased blood pressure; uncoordinated movements; cerebral excitement with incoherent speech, restlessness, disturbed memory, disorientation, delirium, hallucinations; urinary urgency; difficult urination; eye pain; blurred vision; sensitivity to light; dysphagia; great thirst; nausea; vomiting; diarrhea; weakness; convulsions.

Later – Depressed cerebral and neural activity (for example, decreased temperature, depression, drowsiness, stupor, circulatory collapse, fall in blood pressure, coma, and death from centric respiratory paralysis); also, hyperreflexia; decerebrate posturing; pos. Babinski.

Lab – Elevated SGOT and LDH.

EEG – Slow waves, rhythmic burst.

Treatment:

First Aid – Artificial respiration with oxygen; emetic; charcoal (not tannin) or iodide to prevent absorption; antacids can help interfere with absorption.

Medical – Physostigmine 2 mg IV is the best physiological antidote. Gastric lavage; cathartic; keep patient warm and in motion. Catheterize to prevent reabsorption from the urine; repeat antidote as necessary; propanolol for tachyarrhythmias; diazepam for convulsions; chlorpromazine for serious excitation.

Other – Ice bags or sponge baths for fevers. Antidotion with pilocarpine may be tried (but is not effective for CNS symptoms).

References:

3, 6, 7, 9, 13, 14, 103, 107

B

Baptisia tinctoria (L.) R. Br. ex Ait. f.

Fabaceae

Common Names:

Wild indigo, indigo broom, false indigo, American indigo, horsefly weed, yellow indigo, yellow broom

Parts Containing Toxins:

Leaves and roots.

Toxic Constituents – Baptin (phenol glycoside) and baptitoxine or cytisine, sparteine (alkaloids).

Doses:

Therapeutic – Tincture 2-20 drops (0.12-1.23 ml).

Toxic – Powder 30 gm.

Note:

Contraindications – In pregnancy.

Mechanism of Toxicity – Baptitoxine is identical to cytisine, a strong emetic and cathartic. The infusion has neuromuscular depressant effects when administered in large doses.

Toxicity Signs/Symptoms:

Anorexia, vomiting, diarrhea, gastrointesinal spasms; profuse viscid ptyalism; respiration quickens and heart beats stronger until respiratory paralysis causes death.

Treatment:

First Aid – Emesis; activated charcoal;

Medical – Cathartic; if early, do gastric lavage with a liter of potassium permanganate diluted 1:10,000 to inactivate the alkaloid; observe 4 hrs.; IV diazepam for seizures; phenylephrine or dopamine for hypotension.

References:

3, 5, 9, 10, 14, 100, 107, 126

Berberis vulgaris L.   **Berberidaceae**

Common Names:

Barberry, European barberry, pepperidge, sowberry, jaundice berry

Parts Containing Toxins:

Root.

Toxic Constituents – Oxyacanthine, berbamine, berberine (isoquinoline alkaloids); tannins.

Doses:

Therapeutic – Powder 0.32-2.6 gm; tincture 5-60 drops (0.31-3.7 ml). Berberine is well tolerated up to 0.5 gm, equivalent to about 8.0 gm dried root.

Toxic – Berberine sulphate 25-50 mg/kg orally in cats. However, no histopathological changes were found when 0.5 gm/kg berberine sulphate daily was given orally to rats for 6 weeks.

Lethal – Berberine sulphate LD_{50} 14.5 mg/kg IV, 88.5 mg/kg IP, and >1 gm/kg orally in rats; 100 mg/kg orally in cats.

Note:

Contraindications – In pregnancy since it contains the uterine stimulant alkaloids palmatine, berberine, jatorrhizine, and columbamine.

Kinetics – Berberine sulphate given orally to rats is very poorly absorbed.

Mechanism of Toxicity – Berberine causes vasodilation and decreases heart rate through vagal stimulation. It depresses the myocardium in high doses. High doses of berberine also depress respiration, stimulate intestinal smooth muscle and reduce bronchial constriction.

Other – The berries are completely safe.

The closely-related American *Mahonia* spp. contain the same alkaloidal components and have similar effects, so they should also be avoided during pregnancy.

Toxicity Signs/Symptoms:

Mucous membrane irritation, nausea, vomiting; weak pulse, hypotension, heart failure and convulsions; paresthesia.

Treatment:

First Aid – Emesis or gastric lavage; activated charcoal.

Medical – Cathartic; maintain fluid and electrolyte balance. Do baseline hepatic function studies to monitor damage by tannins.

References:

5, 14, 25, 49, 50, 51, 100

Brassica alba (L.) Hooker & Thompson
(= *Sinapis alba* L.);
Brassica juncea (L.) Czern.;
Brassica nigra (L.) Koch   **Brassicaceae**

Common Names:

White mustard; brown mustard, Chinese mustard, Indian mustard ; black mustard, mustard

Parts Containing Toxins:

Seeds; whole plant.

Toxic Constituents – Oil with sinalbin in *B. alba* and sinigrin in *B. juncea* and *B. nigra* (glucosinolates).

Doses:

Therapeutic – Seed oil 3.2-6.5 mg.

Toxic – Seed powder 1 teaspoon.

Note:

Precautions – Do not extend external applications of moist powder in linen beyond 15-30 minutes for adults or 3-5 minutes (5-10 minutes for *B. alba*) for children over age six.

Contraindications – Large doses of seeds internally in pregnancy since they are possibly abortifacient. Internal use should be avoided in gastrointestinal ulcers. External applications should not be made on children under the age of six. Do not use seeds externally or internally if kidney disorders exist. The essential oil of mustard should not be used internally or externally in therapy.

Mechanism of Toxicity – When moistened, sinigrin in the seeds is degraded to allyl isothiocyanate, a potent irritant volatile oil.

Other – Continual use of the whole plants or their leaves as vegetables causes reduced inorganic iodine uptake by the thyroid.

At times all three listed mustard species have been taxonomically identified as belonging to the *Sinapis* genus.

In terms of allyl isothiocyanate release, the potency of these three species varies from *B. juncea* > *B. nigra* > *B. alba.*

The essential oil of horseradish, *Armoracia* spp., is similar in content and effect to mustard essential oil.

Toxicity Signs/Symptoms:

External – [Seeds] The powder can cause burning, vesiculation and inflammation, ulceration, and necrosis of unprotected skin if left in prolonged and/or unprotected contact.

Internal – [Seeds] Vomiting, stomach pain, intestinal inflammation, diarrhea; somnolence, cardiac weakness, breathing difficulties, coma, death.

In dogs, 20-50 mg/kg body weight has produced epithelial hyperplasia and ulcers of the stomach and minor inflammatory foci in the liver.

Chronic – [Whole Plant] Consumption can lead to nontoxic goiter and/or symptoms of hypothyroidism.

Treatment:

First Aid – Emesis; activated charcoal; keep patient warm.

Medical – Gastric lavage if no emesis; cathartic; maintain fluid, pH and electrolyte balance; avoid use of drugs; cardiac massage and artificial respiration with oxygen if necessary.

Other – Demulcents, generous fluids.

References:

2, 3, 6, 10, 12, 14, 25, 100, 105, 106, 107

Bryonia alba L., *Bryonia dioica* Jacquin   Cucurbitaceae

Common Names:

Bryony, white bryony, snakeweed, devil's turnip, bastard turnip, parsnip turnip, tetterberry, wild hops, wild vine, wood vine, ladies' seal

Parts Containing Toxins:

Fresh root; berries.

Toxic Constituents – Bryonin, cucurbitacins (triterpenes), cucurbitacin glycosides.

Doses:

Therapeutic – Root powder 130-650 mg; tincture 1-5 drops (0.06-0.3 ml).

Lethal – Berries 1-15 in children; 40 in adults.

Note:

Contraindications – In cases of hypersensitivity and during pregnancy.

Mechanism of Toxicity – Cucurbitacins are irritants to the gastrointestinal mucosa.

Other – Dermatitis may occur from whole plant contact.

The root is the part employed medicinally.

Toxicity is diminished upon drying the root and when the root is harvested in the spring or autumn.

Toxicity Signs/Symptoms:

Internal – Colic, vomiting, bloody diarrhea, gastroenteritis, kidney irritation, anuriea, cardiac depression with weak, thready pulse, fall of temperature, mydriasis, congestive headaches, dizziness, hyperexcitability, delirium, cold perspiration, spasm, paralysis, and collapse; death.

Nonfatal overdose may cause bronchial irritation with cough, hepatic tenderness, increased urination with vesical tenesmus, tachycardia, drowsiness, cerebral fullness and congestion, jaundice and depressed action of the heart.

External – The fresh root may cause rash, blistering and necrosis.

Treatment:

First Aid – Tannin, strong tea, emetic; use water copiously. Wash for dermatitis.

Medical – Cardiac support when indicated; maintain fluid and electrolyte balance.

Other – Demulcents orally and by enema; keep warm with blankets and by external heat and hot fomentations to the abdomen.

References:

1, 3, 9, 10, 14, 82, 103, 104, 107

C

Cannabis sativa L.   Moraceae

Common Names:

Marijuana, ganja, pot, grass, weed, bhang, Indian hemp

Parts Containing Toxins:

Resin from dried flowering tops.

Toxic Constituents – Tetrahydrocannabinol and others (cannabinoids 15-20%).

Doses:

Therapeutic – Powder 100 mg; tincture 10-20 drops (0.6201.23 ml); fluid extract 1-5 drops (0.06-0.31 ml).

Note:

Contraindications – In pregnancy since tetrahydrocannabinol crosses the human placenta and results in lower birth weight and length. Also, high doses in animals have damaged developing embryos and resulted in birth defects. It also reportedly has oxytocic effects.

Tolerance – Occurs with acute and chronic use.

Kinetics – Readily absorbed; excreted in urine and feces. Stored in lipid tissues, especially CNS, crosses placenta.

Mechanism of Toxicity – Binding to receptor sites in the basal ganglia, hippocampus, cerebral cortex and cerebellum is rapid and reversible, affecting memory, movement and sensation, but leading to no permanent damage. The actions of acetylcholine are reduced in the hippocampus, impairing short-term memory. Low concentration of cannabinoid receptor sites in brain stem control centers for the heart and breathing is probably responsible for lack of fatalities from overdose.

Other – Even moderate marijuana use can induce psychotic symptoms where there is a personal or family history of schizophrenia.

Heavy chronic smoking is associated with respiratory ailments such as laryngitis, bronchitis, sinutsitis, asthma, and rhinopharyngitis.

Driving ability can be impaired for up to 8 hours.

Toxicity Signs/Symptoms:

Acute – Dry mouth and throat, injected conjunctiva; pale and clammy skin, feeble and rapid pulse; impaired short term memory, coordination, tracking, sensory and perceptual skills; giddiness, paranoia, incoherent thought, delusions of grandeur, distorted sense of time, anxiety, panic, confusion, dual personality; illusions, hallucinations; ravenous hunger, weakness, partial anesthesia, decreased temperature, increased systolic blood pressure, disturbed heart function; tremor, spasms, loss of appetite, convulsions; heaviness and numbness of limbs, drowsiness, deep sleep, unsteadiness, staggering, slurred speech, catalepsy, depression, maniacal insanity; collapse. Deaths due to toxic effects are undocumented.

Chronic – Depressed ovarian function, decreased LH and FSH; decreased spermatogenesis and sperm motility, disturbed genital functions; apathy, dullness; impaired judgment, concentration and memory; low interest in appearance, hygiene and diet; loss of ambition, energy and concentration; delirium; diminished REM sleep.

Withdrawal – Irritability, restlessness, nervousness, decreased appetite, weight loss, insomnia; tremor, and chills following heavy, chronic use. Symptoms peak at 30 hours and lasts 4-5 days.

Treatment:

Other - Monitor and keep calm in a safe environment.

References:

4, 6, 8, 9, 10, 13, 83, 84, 103, 104, 107

Capsicum annuum L., *Capsicum frutescens* L.   Solanaceae

Common Names:

Cayenne, African pepper, bird pepper, chili pepper, pod pepper, red pepper

Parts Containing Toxins:

Dried ripe fruit.

Toxic Constituents – Capsaicin (an amide in oleoresin).

Doses:

Therapeutic – Tincture 1/10-10 drops (0.01-0.62 ml).

Toxic – Powder 0.8-1.6 gm.

Note:

Mechanism of Toxicity – Capsaicin is an irritant stimulant of the mucous membranes and skin.

Toxicity Signs/Symptoms:

Internal – [Acute] Increased salivation, sweating, and gastric flow; nausea, vomiting and diarrhea, pain and inflammation of stomach and bowels, colic, hemorrhagic gastritis, dizziness, giddiness, strangury.

Inhaled – Capsaicin causes a dose-dependent bronchoconstriction.

External – Dermatitis.

Internal – [Chronic] Gastritis, kidney damage, liver damage, neurotoxic effects.

Treatment:

First Aid – [Acute Internal] Emesis; activated charcoal.

Medical – [Acute Internal] Gastric lavage; maintain fluid and electrolyte balance; avoid use of drugs.

References:

2, 5, 6, 9, 10, 14, 25, 53, 107, 129, 130, 131

Cassia acutifolia Del.
(= *Cassia alexandrina* P. Mill.
= *Cassia senna* L.);
Cassia angustifolia Vahl;
= *Senna* spp.   Fabaceae

Common Names:

Alexandrian senna; Tinnevelly senna; senna

Parts Containing Toxins:

Fruit pods, leaves.

Toxic Constituents – Sennosides A, B, C, and D (anthraquinone glycosides), sennidines (dianthrones), rhein and aloe-emodin (anthrones)

Doses:

Therapeutic – Powdered leaf 325-1300 mg; tincture 0.5-1.0 tsp (1.85-3.7 ml); fluid extract 5-60 drops (0.62-3.7 ml).

Toxic – LD50 2500 mg/kg senna extract or 4000 mg/kg pure sennosides orally in mice.

Note:

Precaution – Do not use in excess of 8-10 days.

Contraindications – In pregnancy and menstruation, especially menorrhagia and metrorrhagia, and if there are actively inflamed hemorrhoids. Also in intestinal obstruction, abdominal pain of unknown origin, any intestinal inflammation, prolapsed rectum or anus, in kidney dysfunction, and in children under twelve.

Mechanism of Toxicity – Anthraquinone glycosides act as intestinal irritants. This potentiates its action as an emmenagogue and potential abortifacient.

Other – The pods are milder in effect than the leaves.

Use of a standardized extract of senna in controlled, individualized doses during pregnancy may not induce uterine contractions leading to miscarriage. However, aloe-emodin may be genotoxic even in small amounts.

If used while nursing it can cause diarrhea in the infant in some cases.

It may cause a red coloration of the urine. With chronic use the rectal mucosa will have a noticeable black pigmentation.

Bitters increase its purgative effects, while aromatic carminatives can prevent the nausea and cramps.

Loss of potassium from overuse can cause deficiency symptoms and potentiate the cardiotoxic effects of cardiac glycoside medications.

The similar species *Cassia marilandica,Cassia fistula, Cassia obtusifolia* and *Cassia tora* have equivalent effects and contraindications.

Toxicity Signs/Symptoms:

Nausea, flatulence, diarrhea with griping (cramping).

Treatment:

First Aid – Emesis; charcoal.

Medical - Gastric lavage if no emesis.

Other – Demulcents.

References:

3, 9, 100, 101, 103, 104, 106, 107

Catharanthus roseus (L.) G. Don.
(= *Vinca rosea* L.)   Apocynaceae

Common Names:

Madagascar periwinkle

Parts Containing Toxins:

All parts (green or dried).

Toxic Constituents – Vincristine, vinblastine and others (indole alkaloids).

Doses:

Therapeutic – Vincristine 50-150 mcg/kg once weekly; vinblastine 100-500 mcg/kg once weekly.

Note:

Contraindications – In pregnancy due to its abortifacient and teratogenic effects.

Mechanism of Toxicity – Produces granulocytopenia and bone marrow depression through mitotic arrest.

Other – Besides the whole plant toxicity, the isolated alkaloids used in chemotherapy have specific adverse effects as designated below.

Toxicity Signs/Symptoms:

Drowsiness, blurred vision, dry mouth, nausea, ataxia; liver damage, psychosis, hallucinations, convulsions, thirst, alopecia, paresthesia, decreased appetite, stupor, anxiety, depression, confusion, neuropathy, coma, headache, leukopenia; loss of hair, loss of deep tendon reflexes, death.

Vinblastine – In addition to the above, may cause thrombocytopenia, paralytic ileus, urinary retention, bilateral parotid pain, sinus tachycardia, vomiting, anorexia, diarrhea, dermatitis.

Vincristine – In addition to the first list, may cause: fever, neuritic pain, muscle weakness, cranial nerve palsies, peripheral neuritis, severe constipation, hoarseness; ptosis, hyponatremia, double vision, thrombocytopenia, anemia, polyuria.

Treatment:

First Aid – Emesis; activated charcoal.

Medical – Gastric lavage if no emesis; cathartic; supportive care and monitoring; for seizures use IV diazepam.

References:

4, 5, 6, 13, 14, 25, 37, 100

Caulophyllum thalictroides (L.) Michx.
Berberidaceae

Common Names:

Blue cohosh, beechdrops, blue ginseng, papoose root, squaw root

Parts Containing Toxins:

Roots; nonmedicinal berries, leaves and seeds.

Toxic Constituents – 0.033% Methylcytisine, 0.02% baptifoline, 0.012% anagyrine, and magnoflorine (quinolizidine alkaloids) and caulosaponin 0.1% dry weight (saponin) in the rhizome and roots.

Doses:

Therapeutic – Root powder 0.5-1.0 gram; tincture 5-10 drops (0.31-0.62 ml).

Lethal – Methylcytisine LD_{50} 21-22 mg/kg IV and 51 mg/kg IP in mice. Caulosaponin LD_{50} 11.8 mg/kg IV in mice and 20.3 mg/kg IV in rats.

Note:

Contraindications – The root in pregnancy, since it is an emmenogogue, oxytocic, and abortifacient. The component anagyrine is potentially teratogenic.

Mechanism of Toxicity – The root acts as a skin and mucous membrane irritant. Methyl cytisine acts similarly to nicotine on the heart, circulation, respiration and intestinal motility based on *in-vitro* tests, but methylcytisine is 10-25 times less potent.

Other – Circumstantial evidence in one case report associated the use of the root for three weeks prior to delivery with fetal myocardial infarction detected after delivery.

Roasting the seeds reputedly destroys their toxicity.

Nicotine is about 40 times as toxic as methylcytisine in mice.

Toxicity Signs/Symptoms:

Internal – Nausea, vomiting and gastritis, headache, thirst, dilated pupils, muscle weakness, incoordination; cardiovascular collapse and convulsions are usually terminal events.

External – Dermatitis.

Treatment:

First Aid – Emesis and activated charcoal; for contact dermatitis, wash twice with soap and water.

Medical – Cathartic; maintain fluid and electrolyte balance; avoid use of drugs.

References:

5, 6, 11, 14, 25, 89, 90, 91, 100, 104, 106, 107, 108, 132, 133

Cephaelis acuminata Karsten,
Cephaelis ipecacuanha (Brot.) A. Rich.

Rubiaceae

Common Names:

Ipecac, ipecacuanha

Parts Containing Toxins:

Root.

Toxic Constituents – 2% Emetine, cephaeline, psychotrine (isoquinoline alkaloids 2-4%).

Doses:

Therapeutic (Nonemetic) – Powder 16-194 mg; syrup 1-20 drops (0.06 – 1.2 ml); emetine 1 mg/kg body weight for 3-10 days.

Toxic – Powder 1-2 gm.

Note:

Contraindications – In pregnancy; since emetine as an isolated constituent is a uterine stimulant. Avoid using for patients with organic heart disease. Do not use the syrup of ipecac as an emetic when time following toxin consumption is greater than one hour, for children less than 6 months, if there is drowsiness, reduced consciousness, reduced gag reflex, or convulsions, or if vomiting has already occurred or is continuing. Syrup of ipecac should not be used in poisoning from acid or alkali corrosives, volatile hydrocarbons or petroleum distillates, seizure-inducing substances or if sharp objects have been ingested.

Kinetics – Emetine accumulates in the liver, lungs, kidneys and spleen; traces are detectable after 40-60 days.

Mechanism of Toxicity – Emetine causes local irritation and stimulation of medullary emetic center.

Toxicity Signs/Symptoms:

Topically – Reddens and irritates skin and mucosa, producing vesicular and pustular eruptions, ulcerations.

Inhaled – Swollen and inflamed eyes, violent sneezing and heat, dyspnea, nosebleed.

Internal – Wheezing respiration and cough, anxiety and prostration; violent sneezing and spitting blood; nausea, vomiting, diarrhea bilious and mush-like, depressed pulse, dizziness, faintness, headache, languor, diaphoresis, increased secretions, gastroenteritis, mucosal erosion; weakness, aching tenderness, stiffness, tremor, edema; dyspnea; hypotension, precordial pain, tachycardia, cardiac dilatation, cardiac failure; convulsions, shock, and death.

ECG – Flattened and inverted T waves, prolonged Q-T interval.

Treatment:

First Aid – Activated charcoal, give vegetable acids (for example, vinegar, lemon or orange juice) in plenty of water.

Medical – Gastric lavage, cathartic. Balance pH; use plasma expanders for shock; stimulate the heart with belladonna or digitalis; diazepam for spasms; monitor kidney function; mechanical ventilation with oxygen if necessary.

Other – Keep warm and quiet;

References:

6, 7, 9,10, 13, 100, 107, 134, 135, 169

Chelidonium majus L.   **Papaveraceae**

Common Names: Celandine, greater celandine, garden celandine, tetterwort

Parts Containing Toxins: All parts, especially roots.

Toxic Constituents – Chelidonine, protopine, cryptopine (isoquinoline alkaloids), chelerythrine, sanguinarine (benzophenanthridine alkaloids), sparteine (lupinane alkaloid), berberine, tetrahydrocoptisine (protoberberine alkaloids).

Doses:

Therapeutic – Leaf powder 2-4 gm daily; fluid extract 1-2 ml. Root powder 0.5 gm daily; tincture 10-15 drops (0.62-0.93 ml).

Note:

Contraindications – In pregnancy. It contains the animal uterine stimulants chelidonine, sparteine, protopine, chelerythrine and berberine.

Mechanism of Toxicity – The alkaloids berberine, chelerythrine and sanguinarine in celandine inhibit acetylcholinesterase activity.

Toxicity Signs/Symptoms:

Nausea, vomiting, coma; also, burning in the mouth and throat, abdominal pain, bloody diarrhea, bloody urine, stupor, and death.

External – The fresh juice applied to the skin produces rubefaction, inflammation and vesiculation.

Treatment:

First Aid – Charcoal, emesis. For contact dermatitis, wash area twice with soap and water.

Medical – Gastric lavage if no emesis; maintain fluid and electrolyte balance; avoid use of drugs.

References:

1, 6, 7, 9, 14, 25, 92, 100, 107

Chenopodium ambrosioides L.   Chenopodiaceae

Common Names:

Wormseed, feather geranium, goosefoot, Jerusalem oak, Jesuit tea, Mexican tea, American wormseed

Parts Containing Toxins:

Seeds (fruit).

Toxic Constituents – Ascaridole (unsaturated terpene peroxide of volatile oxide); nitrates.

Doses:

Therapeutic – Oil 20 drops (1 ml); fluid extract 1/4-2 tsp (0.93-7.4 ml).

Lethal – Oil 10 mg, 6 drops (0.3 ml) in children, LD_{50} 0.25-0.38 orally in animals.

Note:

Contraindications – In pregnancy due to its emmenagogue and abortifacient effects, or in cases of heart, liver, kidney, stomach or intestinal disease. The oil should not be used internally or externally in therapy.

Mechanism of toxicity – The oil is an irritant to the skin and mucous membranes and a cardiac depressant. Ascaridole is neurotoxic.

Other – Even inhalation of the oil for a short period can induce a headache.

A saline cathartic is given 2 hours after a single dose of the remedy for worms.

Toxicity Signs/Symptoms:

Internal – Burning sensation in throat and mouth, nausea, vomiting; headache, tinnitus, vertigo, drowsiness, sleep, constipation; deafness, decrease in visual acuity, double vision, blindness; decreased respiration, varied heart rate, gastric ulcers, constipation, prostration, spasms, nephritis, decreased blood pressure and CNS activity, spinal cord depression (paralysis) and death by respiratory paralysis. Damage to liver, kidneys, heart, and brain, but especially the CNS.

An extract administered subcutaneously to 30 rats showed carcinogenic activity in 53%

External – Dermatitis.

Treatment:

First Aid – Induce wakefulness with stimulants such as coffee. For contact dermatitis wash with soap and water.

Medical – Gastric lavage if no emesis.

References:

5, 6, 10, 11, 12, 21, 25, 32, 35, 105, 107, 136

Cimicifuga racemosa (L.) Nutt.   Ranunculaceae

Common Names:

Black cohosh, macrotys, black snakeroot, bugbane, bugwort, rattleroot, rattlewort, rattleweed, richweed, squawroot

Parts Containing Toxins:

Roots and rhizome.

Toxic Constituents – Actein, 27-deoxyactein (triterpene glycosides), 15-20% isoferulic acid, cimicifugin, tannins.

Doses:

Therapeutic – Powder 65-1300 mg; tincture 1/2-1 tsp (1.85-3.7 ml); fluid extract 5-30 drops (0.31-1.85 ml).

Toxic – Powder 5 gm

Note:

Precautions – Not to be used for over six months without interuption.

Contraindications – In pregnancy (especially the first trimester) due to its emmenagogue effect.

Kinetics – Excreted by the skin and kidneys.

Mechanism of Toxicity – The roots and rhizome act as a neural sedative and relax nonstriated muscles. The nontoxic component acteina increases peripheral blood flow.

Other – An inconclusive case report noted three nocturnal seizures occurred in a 45-year-old woman over a 3-month period after taking *C. racemosa* with *Vitex agnus-castus* and evening primrose oil capsules for four months. She also consumed one or two beers 24-48 hours prior to each incident.

Toxicity Signs/Symptoms:

General relaxation, injected conjunctive, flushed face, visual dimness, dilated pupils, dizziness or light headedness, nausea, and a dull throbbing, frontal headache, profuse sweating, and reduced heart rate; tremors, decreased blood pressure, vomiting or gastric irritation, prostration; pain in joints and limbs.

Treatment:

First Aid – Emesis; activated charcoal.

Medical – Gastric lavage if no emesis; cathartic; obtain baseline hepatic function studies.

References:

3, 9, 10, 11, 14, 100, 101, 104, 107, 109, 137, 138

Cinchona ledgeriana Moens & Trimen., *Cinchona* spp.

Rubiaceae

Common Names:

Peruvian bark, Jesuits' bark

Parts Containing Toxins:

Bark.

Toxic Constituents – 10% quinoline alkaloids of 5 classes; cinchonine, quinamine, quinin, cusconine and anhydro, e.g., 70% quinine, quinidine

Doses:

Therapeutic – Bark powder 1.0-3.0 gm; tincture 10-60 drops (0.93-3.7 ml); fluid extract 5-30 drops (0.31-1.85 ml); extract (with 15-20% alkaloids) 0.15-0.6 gm; quinine sulphate 65-1300 mg, usual 300 mg); quinidine sulphate 100-300 mg.

Toxic – Quinine over 3 gm; quinidine 1 gm.

Lethal – Quinine 8-15 gm.

Note:

Precautions – Constituents are excreted in breast milk. Never give in continued or excessive doses.

Contraindications – In pregnancy due to its toxic and teratogenic (causes visual and auditory defects, may cause hemolytic anemia) effects and its uterine stimulant, oxytocic and abortifacient effects; in reactive patients (one third of total), or where allergic hypersensitivity or toxicity symptoms for the alkaloids preexist.

Kinetics – Quinine is hydroxylated in the liver and excreted in the urine (5-17% unchanged).

Mechanism of Toxicity – In large doses, cinchona is sedative to the CNS and cardiac plexus.

Other – May potentiate coumarin derivatives as anticoagulants.

Toxicity symptoms described below include those for the quinine and the extract.

Toxicity Signs/Symptoms:

Acute – Headache, nausea, abdominal pains, vomiting and diarrhea; vertigo, tinnitus, visual disturbances such as night blindness, scotomas, mydriasis, color changes; transitory or permanent deafness, depression, renal damage, lowered body tempreature, cold extremities; cardiac arrhythmias, respiration slowed, diaphoresis, skin hot and flushed, then cyanotic; angioedema (face), heart failure and asphyxiation leading to death.

Lab – Hypoprothrombinemia, agranulocytosis.

Hypersensitivity – Purpura, asthma, ventricular tachycardia; possibly erythematous skin rash, itching, thrombocytopenia, nausea, syncope, coma, body temperature and blood pressure falls, death.

Cumulative – Mental confusion and nervous excitement, muscular feebleness, impaired motility, restlessness, wakefulness, eructations, chill and fever paroxysms, perspiration, delirium, tinnitus, deafness, diplopia, photophobia, blurred vision, psychosis.

Quinidine – Besides exhibiting the symptoms of cinchonism listed as cumulative, also causes cardiotoxicity effects including S-A block, A-V block, ventricular arrhythmias or asystole, and ventricular tachycardia.

Treatment:

First Aid – Discontinue use, give strong coffee and charcoal.

Medical – Institute gastric lavage and, if necessary; cathartic; monitor serum potassium; sodium lactate or bicarbonate IV; supportives to the heart and respiration; phenytoin for tachycardia, atropine for bradycardia, lidocaine for arrhythmias, transvenous electrical pacer; norepinephrine; Vit K for hypoprothrombinemia. Remove quinidine with dialysis.

References:

3, 6, 9, 10, 13, 14, 25, 100, 101, 104, 106, 107

Cinnamomum camphora (L.) Siebold   **Lauraceae**

Common Names:

Camphor wood, laurel camphor, cemphire

Parts Containing Toxins:

Wood chips.

Toxic Constituents – Camphor (volatile saturated ketone) 30-50% of volatile oil; safrole, cineole (volatile oxides) in crude camphor oil.

Doses:

Therapeutic – Camphor monobromate 30-300 mg, usually 125 mg.; 10% camphor spirit 1-30 drops (0.06-1.85 ml); camphor water 1-4 tsp (3.7-14.8 ml).

Toxic – Camphor 2-20 grams.

Lethal – Camphor 1 ml in small children, taken as 1 tsp of camphorated oil. Camphor 5-20 gm in adults; 0.005-0.5 gm/kg orally. LD_{50} 5.1 ml/kg orally in animals.

Note:

Contraindications – Camphor in pregnancy due to its emmenagogue, possible abortifacient and feticidal effects. Camphor should not be used on infants or on the face or near the nose of small children under 2 years old. Avoid in epilepsy and fever.

Kinetics – Camphor is rapidly and readily absorbed by the skin, lungs and GI tract. It is metabolized in the liver as glucuronide, which is excreted in the urine and feces. It is also stored in fat and excreted from the lungs.

Mechanism of Toxicity – Camphor acts as a rubefacient, CNS stimulant, and as a local anaesthetic. It neurotoxic effects lead to convulsant activity.

Other – White camphor oil, the most common natural commercial type, is 50% D-camphor and 50% cineole with no safrole.

Most pure commercial camphor is synthetized. It is racemic

mixture, DL-camphor, made from pinene and must be labeled as synthetic. Camphorated oil is 20% camphor in cottonseed oil.

The toxicity described below describes symptoms from excesses of the component camphor but may apply to concentrated alcoholic extracts of the wood or other lipophilic preparations containing camphor in high concentrations.

In infants sudden collapse has occurred by the local application of camphor to their nostrils.

Toxicity Signs/Symptoms:

Internal – Burning pain in esophagus and stomach (gastric ulceration) followed by nausea, emesis, headache, vertigo, mental confusion, feeble intermittent pulse, muscular weakness, mydriasis. Terminal stage involves stupor, delirium; epileptiform convulsions and seizures, collapse; rapid pulse and respiration, tremors, pupilary constriction and veiled vision, incoordination, coma, also death by respiratory failure.

External – Dermatitis.

Treatment:

First Aid – No emesis; activated charcoal. Wash well, if dermal or eye exposure.

Medical – Observe 4 hours, if asymptomatic; gastric lavage; cathartic; opium; avoid oils or alcohol to reduce absorption; IV diazepam for seizures; lipid hemodialysis if severe.

References:

3, 6, 7, 9, 11, 13, 14, 25, 100, 101, 105, 106, 107, 139

Citrullus colocynthis (L.) Schrad.   Cucurbitaceae

Common Names:

Colocynth, bitter apple, bitter gourd, bitter cucumber

Parts Containing Toxins:

Dried pulp of unripe fruit.

Toxic Constituents – Up to 3% E-, J- and L- cucurbitacins and

0.21% alpha-elaterin (glycosides); possibly colocynthin (alkaloid), citrullol (phytosterol glycoside), and/or resins.

Doses:

Therapeutic – Powder 130-325 mg; tincture 1-4 drops (0.06-0.25 ml).

Toxic – Powder 0.6-1.0 gm.

Lethal – Powder 2-6 grams or 1.5 tsp. Alcoholic extract 0.5-3.0 gm/kg acutely or 0.1 gm/kg daily for 3 months orally in mice.

Note:

Precaution – Do not prescribe alone; mitigate with belladonna or hyocyamus.

Contraindications – In pregnancy due to its potent cathartic, mutagenic, and potentially abortifacient effect and when there is abdominal fullness or cardiac palpitation. Nursing mothers should avoid its use, since it is purported to be excreted in breast milk.

Mechanism of Toxicity – The active substances are irritants to the eye and to the nasal and gastrointestinal mucosa.

Toxicity Signs/Symptoms:

Violent emesis and catharsis, bloody stools; vomiting, severe burning and colicky pains; spasms, tenesmus; diuresis, then urinary retention, kidney damage, hemorrhagic cystitis; also weak pulse, muscular weakness, fainting, dizziness,

prostration; fear, raving, delirium; convulsions, paralysis, circulatory collapse, loss of consciousness, death.

Lab – Leukocytosis.

Treatment:

First Aid – Emetic; activated charcoal.

Medical – Gastric lavage if no emesis; maintain fluid and electrolyte balance; avoid use of drugs; opium may be given by mouth or rectum, followed by stimulants.

Other – Demulcents by enema or orally; hot fomentations to the abdomen.

References:

1, 3, 7, 9, 10, 14, 25, 102, 103, 106, 107

Claviceps purpurea (Fries) Tul.   Hypocreaceae

Common Names:

Rye ergot, Secale cornutum, spur, spurred rye, smut rye, ergota

Parts Containing Toxins:

Dried sclerotium grown on Secale .

Toxic Constituents – Ergonovine, ergocornine, ergotamine, ergocryptine, ergosine and ergocristine (indole alkaloids).

Doses:

Therapeutic – Fluid extract 1/2-1 teaspoon (1.85-3.7 ml); extract 520 mg. Ergotamine tartrate 1-2 mg; Ergonovine mal. 0.2 mg.

Toxic – Extract 1.0-3.9 gm.

Lethal – Ergot alkaloids 1 gram in adults; 12 mg in infants; ergotamine tartrate 26 mg oral, 0.5-1.5 mg IM for days.

Note:

Contraindications – In pregnancy due to its uterine stimulant, emmenagogue, oxytocic, and abortifacient effects. Also, avoid using if there is peripheral blood flow disorders, coronary insufficiency, slow GI absorption, pre-existing vascular pathology, hypertonia or severe hypotonia, liver disease, infections or fever.

Kinetics – Half life 2 hours; metabolized by liver, 90% in bile. Peak plasma level is 20 minutes after IM injection.

Mechanism of Toxicity – By alpha-adrenergic blocking and antagonism of 5-hydroxytryptamine (serotonin), it stimulates smooth circular muscles and postganglionic synapses of sympathetic nerves to the uterus, bladder, heart, blood vessels and iris. Large doses cause tetanic spasms.

Toxicity Signs/Symptoms:

Acute – Headache, nausea and vomiting, excessive thirst, itching, diarrhea, dizziness, drowsiness, extreme weakness, muscle pain, fast pulse, dilated pupils, dyspnea, peripheral edema, thrombosis; numbness in fingers, tingling and coldness of skin; muscle twitching, paresthesia, anuria, swollen face, confusion, convulsions; coma and death from respiratory and cardiac failure.

Chronic/Gangrenous – Tingling and formication with reddening, blanching or cyanosis; dilated pupils, dim vision, loss of vision field; aphasia; aching. Vesicles with dark sanguineous exudate over distal extremities leads to gangrene and sloughing. Cataracts are a common result.

Chronic/Spasmodic – Muscle tremors, twitching, or convulsions, clonic spasms leading to tonic spasms; opisthotonus, hunger, extreme weakness, vertigo, tinnitus, numbness, photophobia, violent headaches, mental and physical depression, vomiting and diarrhea, insanity, renal artery spasm, and death.

Treatment:

First Aid – Emesis, activated charcoal; keep the body warm for symptomatic relief.

Medical – Gastric lavage with potassium permanganate and saline cathartics; atropine for abdominal cramps; treat hypotension with fluids; observe 48 hours; sodium nitroprusside or diazoxide for vasoconstriction; IV diazepam or chloral hydrate for seizures; anticoagulant therapy if ischemia; low molecular weight dextran; sodium bicarbonate for acidosis; mechanical ventilation with oxygen if necessary.

Other – Caffeine or coffee for cardiac stimulation.

References:

3, 9, 10, 11, 13, 14, 104, 107

Coffea arabica L.   **Rubiaceae**

Common Names:

Coffee, java, mocha, espresso, joe, caffea

Parts Containing Toxins:

Dried ripe seed.

Toxic Constituents – Caffeine (methylxanthine alkaloid); chlorogenic acid (polyphenolic acid).

Doses:

Therapeutic – Powder 3 gm; infusion 2-8 oz (60-240 ml); caffeine 65-325 mg.

Toxic – Caffeine 1 gm.

Lethal – Caffeine 10 gm, 5.3 gm in child.

Note:

Precautions – Nursing mothers who consume caffeine may have infants with sleeping disorders. Normally safe levels (up to 5 cups per day or 500 mg caffeine) should be avoided in people with cardiac problems, kidney disease, hyperthryoidism, and predisposition to convulsion or anxiety.

Contraindications – In pregnancy in quantities no greater than 3 cups (300 mg) spread over a day, since greater than 600 mg caffeine may produce teratogenic and abortifacient effects.

Kinetics – Half-life 3-6 hours; metabolized in liver, excreted as caffeine in urine and as 1-methyl uric acid and 1-methyl xanthine.

Mechanism of Toxicity – Caffeine is a cerebrospinal stimulant. It also is a muscle and gastric stimulant, a diuretic and a vasodilator.

Other – Caffeine dependence syndrome (caffeinism) is a recognized medical condition consisting of inability to cut down or control use, health problems caused or exacerbated by caffeine, tolerance to caffeine's effects, and withdrawal symptoms.

The following severe acute toxicity symptoms refer especially to the potential effects of toxic amounts of the isolated alkaloid caffeine.

Toxicity Signs/Symptoms:

Acute – Headaches, nausea, vomiting, abdominal spasms, extreme nervousness, restlessness, excitedness, quickened respirations, insomnia, convulsions and cardiac dilatation. Mild delirium, semiconsciousness, fast and irregular pulse, cold extremities and cold clammy perspiration, lowered temperature, anesthesia, cramps, tremors, reeling gait, dimness of vision, increased urination; stiffness, arrhythmic muscle spasms, opisthotonus, arrhythmic tachycardia; death via respiratory arrest or cardiovascular collapse only with extremely high doses of pure caffeine.

Chronic – Hyperacidity, stomach irritation, diarrhea, reduced appetite, indigestion; extreme nervousness, restlessness, exaggerated reflexes, dizziness, cardiac palpitation, anxiety and insomnia, muscular weakness and trembling, atrial premature beats, tachycardia, diarrhea, tinnitus, vertigo, headache, despondency, irritability.

Withdrawal – Headache, fatigue, depression, sleeping disorders.

Treatment:

First Aid – Emesis; activated charcoal.

Medical – Gastric lavage if no emesis; sorbitol; cathartic; carotid sinus massage for paroxysmal atrial tachycardia; monitor urinary output and replace fluids; IV diazepam for seizures.

Other – Demulcents for GI irritation.

References:

3, 6, 9, 10, 13, 14, 100, 107, 140

Colchicum autumnale L.   **Liliaceae**

Common Names:

Meadow saffron, autumn crocus, upstart, naked ladies

Parts Containing Toxins:

Corm and seed, and nonmedicinal leaves and flowers and all parts

Toxic Constituents – Colchicine, demecolcine (tropolone alkaloids).

Doses:

Therapeutic – Seed tincture 10-30 drops 0.62-1.85 ml), fluid extract 1-5 drops (0.06-0.31 ml); corm tincture 5-15 drops (0.31-0.93 ml), fluid extract 1-10 drops (0.06-0.62 ml); colchicine 0.5-1.5 mg every 1-2 hr until pain subsides, not more than 8 mg daily. Do not repeat for 3 days.

Toxic – 125% of therapeutic dose.

Lethal – Seeds 5 gm, 1.0-1.5 gm for child; tincture 15 ml; colchicine 7-200 mg.

Note:

Precautions – Old and weakened patients and those with heart, kidney or gastrointesinal conditions are especially susceptible to toxicity.

Contraindications – In pregnancy due to its mutagenic and feticidal effects, and likewise for nursing mothers. Teratogenic effects can even occur following colchicine consumption by the father before impregnation. It should also be avoided in gastritis and alcoholism.

Kinetics – Metabolized by liver; excreted in bile and urine.

Mechanism of Toxicity – Colchicine converts to oxydicolchicine, which is a cellular irritant, causing congestion and degenerative changes in the GI tract and kidneys, as well as thrombocytopenia with hemorrhage, leukopenia, or liver damage.

Other – Gastrointestinal symptoms persist for ten days.

About 50% of those who are seriously poisoned will die.

Toxicity Signs/Symptoms:

Acute – After 3-6 hours, burning in the throat, difficulty swallowing, thirst. After 12-14 hours nausea, burning skin, vomiting, watery to bloody diarrhea, abdominal pain and cramps, oliguria, fall of blood pressure, weak rapid pulse, anuria, cardiovascular collapse, kidney damage, muscular depression, shock, delirium, convulsions, collapse, coma, ascending paralysis with respiratory failure or circulatory collapse leading to death (possibly during relapse after short remission).

Chronic – Malabsorption, alopecia, kidney damage with oliguria, hepatitis, peripheral neuritis, myopathy, skin alterations, bone marrow damage.

Lab – [Acute] Hematuria, proteinurea, hemoglobin casts in urine; [chronic] pancytopenia, thrombocytopenia with hemorrhages, aplastic anemia, megaloblastic anemia, agranulocytosis, leukopenia.

Treatment:

First Aid – CPR; delay absorption with water, tea, or milk and emesis or activated charcoal.

Medical – Monitor vital signs frequently; gastric lavage if no emesis; saline cathartic; diazepam for convulsion; treat shock; oxygen if necessary; monitor and replace electrolytes and fluid and blood cells; mechanical ventilation with oxygen; atropine for intestinal spasm and opium or morphine for abdominal pain.

Other – Keep patient warm; hot fomentations to the abdomen for abdominal pain and cramps.

References:

1, 3, 6, 7, 9, 10, 12, 13, 14, 30, 34, 37, 103, 104, 106, 107

Conium maculatum L.   Apiaceae

Common Names:

Poison hemlock, hemlock, spotted hemlock, poison fool's parsley, beaver poison

Parts Containing Toxins:

Green full grown fruit, stems and leaves (root is least toxic).

Toxic Constituents – Coniine (piperidine alkaloid) and lamba-coniceine, beta-coniceine, N-methyl coniine, conhydrinone, conhydrine and pseudoconhydrine (alkaloids 0.2-2.5%).

Doses:

Therapeutic – Powder 0.3 gm; fluid extract 1-6 drops (0.06-0.37 ml).

Toxic – Berries 10 gm, leaves 30 gm; coniine 150 mg.

Lethal – Coniine 500 mg.

Note:

Precautions – Children have been poisoned merely by blowing whistles made from its hollow stem.

Contraindications – In pregnancy due to the teratogenic gamma-coniceine.

Mechanism of Toxicity – The alkaloids stimulate and then paralyse nicotinic receptors of peripheral ganglia; peripheral motor and sensory endings are depressed in large doses.

Other – Drying and cooking are said to diminish the extreme toxicity.

The related nonmedicinal species *Cicuta maculata*, or water hemlock, is also extremely poisonous but this is due to the compound cicutoxin.

Toxicity Signs/Symptoms:

Vomiting and diarrhea, burning mouth, scratchy throat, inflammation of GI tract and congestion of abdominal organs; salivation, loss of appetite, lack of coordination, staggering gait, rolling eyes, visual disorders. Nausea, mental confusion, convulsions, prostration, palpebral ptosis, slow feeble pulse, hypotension, difficult articulation, dilated pupils, fever, deglutination, muscular weakness followed by ascending paralysis; nervousness, trembling, ataxia, loss of orientation; intellect remains clear and intact; the urine has a "mousy" odor; also violent stomach pain, coldness of extremities, cyanosis, numbness; and dyspnea with respiratory failure and cardiovascular collapse leading to death.

Treatment:

First Aid – CPR, emesis, then activated charcoal; coffee.

Medical – Gastric lavage with potassium permanganate or tannins; saline cathartic, fluids administered freely; plasma volume expanders for shock, sodium bicarbinate for acidosis; mechanical ventilation with oxygen if necessary; IV diazepam for seizures; phenylephrine or dopamine for hypotension.

Other – Nux vomica for respiratory emergencies; keep head low and body warm.

References:

1, 3, 6, 7, 9, 10, 12, 14, 34, 103, 104, 107, 141

Convallaria majalis L.   **Liliaceae**

Common Names:

Lily-of-the-valley, May lily, May bells

Parts Containing Toxins:

Whole herb, flowers, roots, fruit (green and dried).

Toxic Constituents – Convallarin, convallamarin, and convallotoxin (steroid glycosides); about 40 other cardenolides have been isolated.

Doses:

Therapeutic – Tincture 5-20 drops (0.31-1.23 ml); fluid extract 5-10 drops (0.31-0.62 ml).

Note:

Precautions – Effects are enhanced by quinidine, calcium, and lowering of potassium levels by diuretics, laxatives and glucocorticoids.

Contraindications – Potassium deficiency and digitalis glycoside therapy.

Kinetics – Only about 10% of the active glycosides are absorbed, and 16% of these undergo protein binding. Elimination is through the kidneys and liver.

Mechanism of Toxicity – It has a similar cardiac and gastric action to *Digitalis* spp., but noncumulative and more rapid acting. It also produces a positive inotropic effect on the myocardium.

Other – A dose of dry powdered herb of 1/10 gram equals 12 digitalis units in potency. Its toxicity occurs more rapidly than it does for digitalis.

Dermatitis may occur with contact of fresh plant.

Toxicity Signs/Symptoms:

Nausea, vomiting, headache, violent purging, cardiac arrhythmias, increased blood pressure, restlessness, trembling; mental confusion, stupor, disordered perception of color, extreme weakness, depression, collapse of circulation, death.

Treatment:

First Aid – Emesis; activated charcoal.

Medical – Gastric lavage if no emesis; cathartic; phenytoin; transvenous electrical pacer. Atropine 0.6 mg IV adults or 0.05 mg/kg/dose IV children. Monitor and treat serum potassium imbalance with Kayeralate (R) or glucose/insulin for hyperkalemia.

References:

1, 5, 7, 8, 10, 12, 14, 93, 106, 107

Copaiba langsdorffii (Desfontaines) O. Kuntze, *Copaiba* spp.   Fabaceae

Common Names:

Balsam of copaiba, copaiva, capivi, balsam of capivi

Parts Containing Toxins:

Oleoresin.

Toxic Constituents – 40-75% Volatile oil with copaene and 35% resin with diterpenoid oleoresins.

Doses:

Therapeutic – Oleoresin 5-30 drops (0.3–1.8 ml).

Toxic – Resin 5 gm.

Note:

Precaution – Avoid in acute gonococcal urinary tract infections.

Mechanism of Toxicity – The resin is irritating to the mucosa.

Other – The oleoresin is soluble in oil, partially soluble in alcohol, and insoluble in water.

Toxicity Signs/Symptoms:

Internal – Nausea and vomiting, stomach pains, eructations, impaired digestion, gastroenteritis; shivers, tremors, pains in the groin, blood in the urine, insomnia;

transient rash with formication and pruritis or erythematous, urticarial or bullous outbreak.

External – Contact dermatitis with erythema, urticaria, petechias, rashes that may leave brown spots.

Treatment:

(See Treatment section under Explanation of Format.)

References:

3, 9, 107

Crocus sativus L.   Iridaceae

Common Names:

Saffron, autumn crocus, Spanish saffron

Parts Containing Toxins:

Stigma and styles.

Toxic Constituents – Alpha-crocetin, crocin (carotenoids), picrocrocin (volatile glycoside).

Doses:

Therapeutic – 0.6-1.5 grams.

Toxic – 5.0 gm.

Lethal – 20 gm (in one case as little as 1.5 gm has been reported as lethal).

Note:

Contraindications – In pregnancy since it has been used as an emmenagogue and is a human abortifacient at a 10 gm dose. Death has occurred after attempted abortion.

Mechanism of action – Thrombocytopenia and hypothrombinemia lead to bleeding tendencies.

Other – In animal tests saffron stigma have shown no significant toxicity.

Toxicity Signs/Symptoms:

Flushing, purpura, epistasis, bleeding from the lips and eyelids, dizziness, numbness, vertigo, vomiting; bradycardia and stupor, profuse metrorrhagia, bloody diarrhea, blood in the urine, death.

Treatment:

First Aid – CPR; emesis; activated charcoal.

Medical – Gastric lavage if no emesis; cathartic.

References:

5, 14, 25, 100, 103, 104, 106, 174

Croton tiglium L.   Euphorbiaceae

Common Names:

Croton oil, oleum tiglii

Parts Containing Toxins:

Oil from seeds.

Toxic Constituents – Phorbols (terpenoids) from nonvolatile oil; (Crotin, a toxic albuminous substance, is not extracted in the oil).

Doses:

Therapeutic – Oil 1-2 drops (0.06-0.12 ml) in emulsion or pill form.

Note:

Contraindications – In pregnancy due to its abortifacient effect. Do not use in children, GI, hemorrhoidal, peritoneal or renal irritation, great prostration or weakness.

Mechanism of Toxicity – The fixed oil is an irritant to skin and mucous membranes.

Toxicity Signs/Symptoms:

Internal – Burning pain in mouth and stomach, GI inflammation, tenesmus, vomiting, watery or bloody diarrhea, pallor, collapse, fall of blood pressure, tachycardia, coma, death.

External – Vesicles, pustules, and diarrhea.

Treatment:

First Aid – Decrease absorption and reduce GI irritation with tap water or milk; remove it by emesis .

Medical – Gastric lavage if no emesis; maintain hydration; opiates for pain and to restrain purgation; Atropine will reduce GI secretions. If collapse threatens, external heat and heart stimulants (subcutaneous) should be given.

Other – Demulcents for mucosal irritability.

References:

1, 3, 7, 9, 10, 14, 25

Cullen corylifolia (L.) Medicus.
(= *Psoralea corylifolia* L.)   Euphorbiaceae

Common Names:

Scurfy pea

Parts Containing Toxins:

Seeds.

Toxic Constituents – Psoralens (furanocoumarins).

Doses:

No ranges given.

Note:

> **Contraindications** – In pregnancy due to its abortifacient effect. Prolonged exposure to sunlight should be avoided.

> **Mechanism of Action** – Psoralens in this plant are photosensitizing through free radical formation by light activation.

Toxicity Signs/Symptoms:

> Nausea, vomiting, malaise, headache, purging.

Treatment:

> (See Treatment section under Explanation of Format.)

References:

> 100

Cytisus scoparius (L.) Link
(= *Sarothamnus scoparius* (L.) Wimm. ex Koch)
Fabaceae

Common Names:

> Broom tops, Scotch broom, link, Irish broom

Parts Containing Toxins:

> Dried tops collected before flowering, flowers, seeds.

> **Toxic Constituents** – Up to 1.5% sparteine, isosparteine (quinolizidine alkaloids) in tops; more than 2% tyramine (biogenic amine) in flowers.

Doses:

> **Therapeutic** – Powder 320-970 mg; tincture 10-30 drops (0.62-1.85 ml). Sparteine sulphate 3.24-32.4 mg.

> **Toxic** – Sparteine > 300 mg

> **Lethal** – Sparteine LD_{50} 42-44 mg/kg IP in rats.

Note:

> **Precaution** – No more than 1/6 grain of sparteine sulphate should be used for the initial dosage.

Contraindication – In pregnancy due to its oxytocic and potentially abortifacient effects. Avoid in hypertension and A-V block.

Kinetics – From 6-10% of Caucasions but less than 1% of Orientals lack the enzyme cytochrome P_{450} IID6 that induces the oxidation of sparteine. These poor metabolisers of sparteine are more susceptible to its adverse effects.

Mechanism of Toxicity – Small doses stimulate the heart, but do not affect respiration; large doses suppress cardiac contractility and paralyze respiratory centers. Sparteine has negative inotropic and chronotropic effects. Tyramine is an indirect sympathomimetic.

Other – Avoid the consumption of extracts of flowers with monoamine oxidase inhibitors due to the flowers' tyramine content which may lead to a hypertensive crisis.

No deaths have been proven to be due to the herb, but sparteine overdose has proven fatal.

The following symptoms include those from excesses of the herb or the alkaloid sparteine

Toxicity Signs/Symptoms:

Nausea, vomiting, diarrhea, dizziness, sweating, trembling, muscular incoordination; headache, anorexia, cramps, vertigo; dilated pupils, ocular palsy, diplopia and blurred vision; heaviness of limbs, prickling in the extremities, sleepiness; palpitations, cardiac arrhythmia, decreased pulse rate; tonic and clonic convulsions, paralysis of motor and respiratory centers; secondary depression and general debility; death by asphyxia.

Treatment:

First Aid – CPR; emesis; activated charcoal.

Medical – Gastric lavage if no emesis; cathartic; diazepam or clhorpromazine for spasms; mechanican ventilation with oxygen for asphyxiation.

References:

3, 5, 6, 7, 9, 10, 12, 14, 25, 52, 101, 104, 106, 107, 142, 143

D

Datura stramonium L.; *Datura* spp.   **Solanaceae**

Common Names:

Jimson weed, Jamestown weed, thornapple, devil's apple, devil's trumpet, mad-apple, stinkweed; angel's trumpet

Parts Containing Toxins:

Leaves, seeds, root, all parts.

Toxic Constituents – Hyoscyamine, hyoscine also called scopolamine, and atropine (tropane alkaloids, 0.2-0.4% in leaves, 0.4% in seeds).

Doses:

Therapeutic – Leaf powder 6.5-64.8 mg; tincture 1/2-8 drops (0.03-0.48 ml); fluid extract 1/2-3 drops (0.03–0.18 ml).

(See *Atropa belladonna* for alkaloid dosages.)

Toxic – Powder 5 grains.

Lethal – Fresh leaf 4-5 grams in children, dry leaf powder 15-100 gm in adults; seeds 15-25 gm; atropine 100 mg.

Note:

Precautions – Avoid in patients with urine retention and cororary sclerosis.

Contraindications – In glaucoma, bowel obstruction, pyloric stenosis, enlarged prostate, acute pulmonary edema, tachyarrhythmias.

Kinetics – Decreased GI motility delays absorption. Symptoms appear after several minutes or hours.

Mechanism of Toxicity – The three alkaloids listed are anticholinergic by competitive inhibition of acetylcholine at the neuroreceptor site. Initially CNS stimulation occurs but is followed by exhaustion and sleep.

Other – *Datura metel* leaf is a common ingredient in imported herbal cigarettes from India.

Other American species have the same components and similar effects such as *Datura innoxia* in the Southwest and *Datura candida* (or *Brugmansia candida*) in Hawaii.

Due to their supposed euphoric action, abuse and overdose do occur.

Toxicity Signs/Symptoms:

Dilated pupils, dry red skin and dry mucous membranes, weak rapid pulse; nausea, thirst, vomiting, impaired vision, staggering, dizziness, incoherence, confusion, disorientation, combativeness, restlessness, agitation, giddiness, visual and auditory hallucinations; delirium with laughter, loquacity and violence; drowsiness, stupor, lethargy, loss of consciousness; constipation, inability to urinate, convulsions, circulatory collapse prior to death.

Lab – Elevated liver enzymes and prothrombin times.

Treatment:

First Aid – Emetic; charcoal.

Medical – Gastric lavage; physostigmine 0.5-2 mg IV over 2-5 minutes or IM for severe hallucinations, repeat antidote after 20 minutes as necessary up to 4 doses; mechanical ventilation with oxygen for respiratory distress; catheterize to prevent reabsorption; cathartic; chlorpromazein for severe excitation; diazepam for convulsions; propanolol for arrhythmias if hemodynamic compromise is detected; blood to pH 7.

Other – Keep in motion; ice bags and sponge baths for fevers in children.

References:

3, 5, 6, 7, 8, 9, 10, 12, 13, 14, 18, 32, 103, 106, 107, 144, 145, 146, 147

Delphinium ajacis L.,
 Delphinium consolida L.   **Ranunculaceae**

Common Names:

Larkspur, lark's claw, knight's spur, staggerweed

Parts Containing Toxins:

Entire plant, including roots and seeds.

Toxic Constituents – Delphinine and ajacine (steroidal alkaloids); delphinidine.

Doses:

Therapeutic – For topical use only.

Lethal – Seed oil LD_{50} in mice was 833-1308 (usual 1046) mg/kg IP, equivalent to 1.25 mg/kg of the total alkaloids.

Note:

Precautions – May be toxic if absorbed through abraded skin.

Mechanism of Toxicity – The alkaloids lead to initial excitation followed by a depression of activity, sensitivity, muscular tone, and respiration.

Other – The plants are more potent in the spring.

Toxicity Signs/Symptoms:

Restlessness, stiffness, muscular twitching, rapid and difficult breathing, bloating, nausea, constipation, weak and rapid pulse and general bodily weakness; bradycardia, depression, convulsions, vomiting, stomach upset, burning sensation of the mouth and skin, hypotension, intense headache, blurred vision; also, death in 1-6 hours by cardiac arrest or respiratory paralysis.

Treatment:

First Aid – [Internal] Emesis; activated charcoal.

Medical – [Internal] Gastric lavage if no emesis; cathartic; transvenous electrical pacer.

First Aid – [External] For contact dermatitis wash twice with soap and water and prevent from scratching.

Medical – [External] Corticosteroids, diphenhydramine.

References:

7, 8, 12, 14, 94, 103, 104, 106, 107

Delphinium staphisagria L.   Ranunculaceae

Common Names:

Stavesacre, lousewort

Parts Containing Toxins:

Dried ripened seed.

Toxic Constituents – Delphinine, aconitine (steroid alkaloids).

Doses:

Therapeutic – Powder 65-130 mg; tincture 1-3 drops (0.06-0.18 ml).

Toxic – Seeds 2 tsp.

Note:

Other – Its topical use as a parasiticide has proven fatal for a child.

Toxicity Signs/Symptoms:

Internal – Nausea, vomiting, inflamed throat, salivation, gastroenteritis; itching skin, urinary and stool urgencey; convulsions, depression of the spinal centers and medulla, loss of sensation and motion, slow pulse and breathing, cardiac or respiratory paralysis leading to death.

External – Reddening, inflammation, eczema.

Treatment:

First Aid – Emetic; activated charcoal.

Medical – Gastric lavage if no emesis; saline cathartic; opiates for pain; diazepam for spasms; sodium bicarbinate for acidosis; mechanical ventilation with oxygen if necessary.

Other – Demulcents orally and by enema; keep patient warm; hot fomentations to abdomen.

References:

1, 3, 6, 7, 8, 9, 10, 103, 107

Digitalis lanata Ehrh.;
Digitalis purpurea L.   **Scrophulariaceae**

Common Names:

Grecian foxglove; purple foxglove, foxglove, witch's gloves, fairy's glove, fairy caps, fairy thimples

Parts Containing Toxins:

Leaves, seeds, flowers.

Toxic Constituents – Digitoxin, gitoxin, gitaloxin, digitonin from *D. purpurea*; digoxin, lanatosides from *D. lanata* (steroida glycosides, at least another dozen similar cardenolides have been isolated from each species).

Doses:

Therapeutic – Powder 32.4- 97.2 mg; tincture 1-15 drops (0.06-0.93 ml); digoxin 0.125-0.5 mg; digitoxin 0.05-0.2 mg.

Toxic – Powder 520 mg.

Lethal – Powder 2 grams.

Note:

Precautions – The simultaneous use of sympthomimetics, methyxanthines, phosphodiesterase inhibitors, or quinidine increases the risk of arrhythmias.

Contraindications – In second or third degree atrioventricular blocks, hypercalcemia, hypertrophic cardiomyopathy, carotid sinus syndrome, ventricular tachycardia, thoracic aortic aneurysm and Wolff-Parkinson-White syndrome.

Kinetics – The differences between the major cardioactive components are great. For digoxin, absorption is from 60-80% with a half-life of about 40 hours and protein binding about

20%. The duration lasts from 4-8 days, and it is excreted by the kidneys. Digitoxin, on the other hand, has an absorption of 95-100% and a half-life of about 200 hours with 90-97% protein binding. The duration of its effects is from 10-21 days, and it is excreted through the liver and kidneys.

Mechanism of Toxicity – In excessive doses it increases the irritability of ventricular muscle, causing extrasystoles, then ventricular tachycardia, then ventricular fibrillation.

Other – Potassium loss increases toxicity; calcium increase also potentiates activity, as does *Rauvolfia serpentina* (reserpine).

Toxicity Signs/Symptoms:

Loss of appetite, headache, nausea and vomiting, diarrhea; bloody stool, abdominal pain, fatigue, trigeminal neuralgia, aberrant color vision (seeing all objects as blue), blurred vision, loss of visual acuity, exophthalmos, delirium, lethargy, depression; sinus bradycardia, premature depolarizations; slow, irregular or dicrotic pulse, stomach disorders, confusion, aphasia, hallucinations, skin rash; drowsiness, tremor, convulsions, fall in blood pressure, cardiac arrhythmias of almost any type, conduction blocks, coma, often after ventricular tachycardia or A-V junctional tachycardia; death from ventricular fibrillation or asphyxiation.

ECG – Heart block, ventricular premature beats, depressed ST segment, lengthened P-R interval; ventricular, nodal or atrial tachycardia.

Age – In infants, cardiac arrhythmias are most common.

In children, CNS depression may occur.

Elderly patients may have bizarre mental symptoms.

Lab – Serum potassium is elevated in acute toxicity, but is lowered in chronic use. Eosinophilia is noted.

Treatment:

First Aid – CPR, emesis followed with activated charcoal.

Medical – Gastric lavage if no emesis; cathartic; digoxin-specific Fab antibody fragments, cholestyramine orally prevents absorption and reduces half-life, and/or hemoperfusion to eliminate glycosides. Atropine (0.01 mg/kg IV) to increase heart rate for partial atrioventricular block; lidocaine without epinephrine for ventricular extrsystole; force fluids (2-3 liters) if kidney function is normal; phenytoin as an antirrhythmic; transvenous electrical pacer; treat hypokalemia, but potassium contraindicated if there is an A-V block.

Other – Aconite or tincture of opium; fluid extract senega given as 10 drops in a tablespoon of water.

References:

1, 3, 4, 6, 8, 9, 10, 12, 13, 14, 93, 103, 107

Dioscorea villosa L.   **Dioscoreaceae**

Common Names:

Wild yam, colic root, rheumatism root

Parts Containing Toxins:

Root.

Toxic Constituents – Dioscin (saponin).

Doses:

Therapeutic – Powder 1.9-3.9 gm.

Note:

Mechanism of Toxicity – Its saponins act as gastrointestinal irritants.

Other – The aglycone of dioscin is diosgenin. Diosgenin has been used in pharmaceutical manufacturing as a precursor for steroidal hormones.

Toxicity Signs/Symptoms:

Nausea, vomiting, diarrhea.

Treatment:

(See Treatment section under Explanation of Format.)

References:

5, 6, 107

Dryopteris filix-mas   Polypodiaceae

Common Names:

Male fern, aspidium, sweet brake, knotty brake

Parts Containing Toxins:

Whole herb.

Toxic Constituents – 2% Filicin, filicinic acid (acylphloroglucinoles).

Doses:

Therapeutic– Oleoresin 2-5 grams given only once; fluid extract 1/2-1 tsp (1.9-3.7 ml).

Note:

Contraindications – In pregnancy due to its abortifacient effect. Also avoid in anemia, gastrointestinal ulceration, diabetes, impaired cardiac, hepatic or renal function, in old or debilitated patients, in children under age 4, and in nursing mothers.

Mechanism of Toxicity – The gastrointestinal irritants are safe in small doses unless given with fixed oils, fats or alcohol which increase absorption. Liver, heart, kidney, and CNS damage occur and can lead to permanent damage inculding paralysis and blindness.

Other – Do not repeat internal doses for several weeks.

Toxicity Signs/Symptoms:

Headaches, vertigo, diarrhea, dyspnea, xanthopsia, transient blindness, loss of reflexes, cyanosis, tremors, cramps; fainting, delirium, psychosis, convulsions and coma, death due to cardiac or respiratory failure.

Visual and aural disturbances, asthenia and bradycardia may persist for some time after emergency is past.

Lab – Albuminuria, bilirubinuria.

Treatment:

> **First Aid** – Emetic.
>
> **Medical** – Gastric lavage and follow with epsom salt cathartic.
>
> **Other** – Colonic irrigation; keep patient warm; caffeine, ammonia, or nux vomica for stimulation if cardiac failure is involved.

References:

> 3, 5, 9, 25, 100, 107

E

Ecballium elaterium (L.) A. Rich   **Cucurbitaceae**

Common Names:

> Squirting cucumber, elaterium, wild cucumber, wild balsam-apple

Parts ContainingToxins:

> Juice of unripe fruit.
>
> **Toxic Constituents** – Elaterin or cucurbitacins (tetracyclic triterpene glycosides)

Doses:

> **Therapeutic** – Elaterin 3-5 mg.

Note:

> **Contraindications** – Do not use in the weak or feeble subjects.
>
> **Mechanism of Toxicity** – The juice acts by irritation causing severe dermitis with inflammation and edema on the skin or gastrointestinal inflammation internally.

Toxicity Signs/Symptoms:

> Violent vomiting, cramps, gastroenteritis, watery purgation,

tachycardia, neurotoxicity, anuria, renal insufficiency, uremia, death from cardiorespiratory failure.

Treatment:

First Aid – Empty stomach.

Medical – Opiates for pain.

Other - Give demulcents by mouth and enema. Maintain body heat by external warmth (hot fomentations to the abdomen). Brandy or whiskey.

References:

9, 10, 148

Ephedra equisetina Bunge, *Ephedra sinica* Stapf.   **Ephedraceae**

Common Names:

Chinese ephedra, Chinese jointfir, ma huang

Parts Containing Toxins:

Stems and twigs; roots and fruits to some extent.

Toxic Constituents – Ephedrine, pseudoephedrine (2-aminophenylpropane alkaloids).

Doses:

Therapeutic – Tincture (1:4) 6-8 ml; ephedrine sulfate 15-30 mg every 3-4 hours.

Toxic – Ephedrine > 300 mg in one day.

Lethal – Ephedrine 1-2 gm.

Note:

Precautions – Use inadvisable in anorexic, insomniac, or suicidal. Combining ephedrine with caffeine enhances toxic potential.

Contraindications – In pregnancy since it is an animal uterine stimulant. Avoid in enlarged prostate, in organic heart disease, hypertension, diabetes, anxiety or restlessness, closed-angle glaucoma, impaired cerebral circulation, pheochromocytoma, and hyperthyroidism.

Mechanism of Toxicity – The alkaloid ephedrine is sympathomimetic but less potent, slower and longer-acting than epinephrine. It displaces norepinephrine from cytoplasmic mobile pool, acting both as a beta- and alpha-agonist. When used chronically, several of the alkaloids act as a substrate in forming stones in the urinary tract.

Other – This herb exhibits marked tachyphylaxis (aucte tolerance with frequent use).

Do not take with with monoamine oxidase inhibitors, ergot alkaloids, cardiac glycosides, halothane or guanethidine.

The similar species from Europe and Asia, *Ephedra distachya*, *Ephedra gerardiana*, and *Ephedra intermedia*, have equivalent effects and the same contraindications.

The following symptoms apply to the use of the plant and/or its alkaloid ephedrine.

Toxicity Signs/Symptoms:

Acute – CNS effects including nausea, vomiting, sweating, vertigo, tremor, throbbing headache; tenseness, nervousness, apprehension, motor restlessness, irritability, and insomnia; dilated pupils, elevated temperature, hypertension, urinary retention, heart palpitation and tachycardia; flushing skin, dizziness, tingling and numbing of extremities; fear, anxiety, psychosis; weakness; myocardial infarction, stroke, seizures, convulsions, cardiac failure or asphyxiation leading to death.

Chronic – Kidney stone formation.

Treatment:

First Aid – Emesis; activated charcoal.

Medical – Gastric lavage with potassium permanganate if no emesis; cathartic; monitor ECG; monitor vital signs, urinary output and serum electrolytes; sodium bicarbonate for acidosis; propranolol for severe palpitations; IV diazepam for seizures; lidocaine for atrial premature beats or ventricular tachycardias;

nitroprusside or phentolamine for hypertensive crises; mechanical ventilation with oxygen if necessary.

Other – Rest, quiet, recumbency, reassurance; supportive therapy for mild toxicities.

References:

4, 5, 6, 7, 13, 14, 25, 56, 57, 58, 100, 106, 107

Equisetum spp.   Equisetaceae

Common Names:

Horsetail, scouring rush, shavegrass

Parts Containing Toxins:

Fresh whole plant.

Toxic Constituents – Articulatin; silicic acid, traces of nicotine (pyridine alkaloid).

Doses:

Therapeutic – Powder < 2.0 gm.

Note:

Precautions – Powdered form is not recommended for children or for prolonged use due to its high silica content.

Contraindications – In those with hypertensive disease, cardiovascular, cardiac, or renal problems. *Equisetum arvense* and *Equisetum hyemale* should be avoided in pregnancy.

Mechanism of Toxicity – Thiamine deficiency may occur with chronic exposure to large amounts of *Equisetum* containing the thiaminase component articulatin.

Other – *Equisetum palustre* contains the toxic alkaloid palustrine.

Toxicity Signs/Symptoms:

Chronic – Thiamine deficiency symptoms (for example, peripheral neuropathy, cardiac, and acute cerebral symptoms).

In animals, muscular weakness, ataxia, weight loss,

abnormal pulse rate, cold extremities, and fever have resulted after chronic ingestion of large quantities.

Treatment:

First Aid – [Acute] Emesis; activated charcoal.

Medical – [Acute] Gastric lavage if no emesis; cathartic.

Medical – [Chronic] Thiamine injection and supplementation.

References:

5, 6, 12, 14, 95, 96, 97, 98, 100, 104, 107

Erythroxylon coca Lamarck   **Erythroxylaceae**

Common Names:

Coca, cuca

Parts Containing Toxins:

Leaves.

Toxic Constituents – Cocaine (tropane alkaloid).

Doses:

Therapeutic – Powdered leaf 3.89-15.6 gm; fluid extract 5-30 drops (0.31-1.85 ml); cocaine HCl 8.1-64.8 mg (usual 16.2 mg, and never more as an initial dose).

Lethal – Cocaine as little as 20-30 mg (on mucous membrane of a susceptible individual).

Note:

Contraindications – In pregnancy due to its emmenagogue action of the leaves which may abort fetus. It is also embrotoxic and passes into mother's milk. The abuse of cocaine in pregnancy and while nursing, as at all times, must be avoided to prevent dependency of the newborn and the mother on this drug.

Kinetics – Half-life 1 hour; degraded by plasma esterases and hepatic enzymes.

Mechanism of Toxicity – Acts as an indirect sympathomimetic in the adrenergic interneuronal synapses by blocking cellular uptake of norepinephine. It causes cardiovascular and central nervous system stimulation, followed by depression.

Other – The toxicity symptoms below refer to the abuse of cocaine, not to the local anesthetic application of cocaine to the eye or the medicinal use of coca leaves.

Toxicity Signs/Symptoms:

Acute – CNS stimulation including hyperreflexia, tremors, delusions, hallucinations, paranoia; followed by depression, excitement, confusion, nausea and vomiting, sweating and dryness of mouth, headache, cardiac arrhythmias, tachycardia, hypertension, sensation of heat; psychosis, mydriasis and exophthalmos, mental and nervous excitement, Cheyne-Stokes respiration, trembling, tremors, hyperthermia, hypotension and shock, leading to convulsions and unconsciousness; death due to cardiovascular compression and asphyxia.

Chronic – Emotional liability, loss of appetite, "startle" reactions, dyskinesias, postural abnormalities, mental impairment, loss of memory, delusions, insomnia, withdrawal from social contacts, digestive problems, emaciation,

muscular twitching; sensation of bugs under skin; perforated or ulcerated nasal septum.

Withdrawal – Cocaine cravings, prolonged sleep, fatigue, lassitude, hyperphagia, depression.

Treatment:

First Aid – [Acute] Charcoal if ingested orally (unlikely).

Medical – [Acute] Artificial airway to establish respirations; do not treat the initial hypertension; Trendelenberg position and fluid for hypotension; prevent hyperthermia by keeping cool and calm; IV diazepam for seizures or psychosis; dopamine or levarterenal for hypotension; lidocaine, propranolol, phenytoin, or verapamil for arrhythmias.

Other – [Acute] Recumbent posture, fresh air, supportive care; strong coffee by mouth or rectum; brandy.

References:

4, 9, 13, 14, 25, 103, 107

Euonymous atropurpureus Jacquin   Celastraceae

Common Names:

Wahoo, Indian arrow-wood, burning bush, spindle tree, gadrose, gatten, pigwood, skewerwood, spindletree

Parts Containing Toxins:

Seeds and fruit; leaves, bark.

Toxic Constituents – Furan-a-carboxylic acid; d-phenyl-glucosone (sterol glucoside); euatroside, euatromonoside (steroid glycosides).

Doses:

Therapeutic – Bark powder 0.3-3.9 gm; tincture 1-3 tsp (3.7-11.1 ml); fluid extract 3-15 drops (0.18-0.93).

Note:

The seeds are the most poisonous.

The bark and root bark are the parts used medicinally.

Toxicity Signs/Symptoms:

Nausea, vomiting, diarrhea, weakness, chills, coma or convulsions, mental symptoms.

Treatment:

First Aid – Emesis; activated charcoal.

Medical – Gastric lavage if no emesis; saline cathartic; maintain fluid and electrolyte balance; plasma volume expander; hemoperfusion to eliminate glycosides; cholestyramine to interupt enterohepatic circulation; mechanical ventilation with oxygen if necessary; avoid the use of drugs if possible.

Other – Keep quiet and warm.

References:

1, 3, 12, 14, 107

Eupatorium perfoliatum L.   Asteraceae

Common Names:

Boneset, thoroughwort, Indian sage, ague weed, crosswort, feverwort, vegetable antimony, sweating plant

Parts Containing Toxins:

Leaves and tops.

Toxic Constituents – Eupatorin (flavone glycoside); eupafolin and others (sesquiterpene lactones).

Doses:

Therapeutic – Powder 2-4 gm; tincture 15-40 drops (0.93-2.47 ml).

Toxic – Over 4 oz (120 ml) of the hot infusion prepared with 1 oz (31.1 gm) herb in 1 pt (475 ml) boiling water.

Note:

Mechanism of Toxicity – Eupatorin is cytotoxic and a strong emetic, while the bitter components acts as gastrointestinal irritants. The lactones may cause skin sensitization.

Other – Though many *Eupatorium* spp., including the medicinal *Eupatorium purpureum* (gravel root), contain hepatotoxic pyrrolizidine alkaloids, *E. perfoliatum* does not appear to have these compounds.

The nonmedical *Eupatorium rugosum* (richweed) that contains the toxin tremetol is difficult to distinguish from *E. perfoliatum*. Though tremetol yield is greatly reduced by drying, a risk of poisoning exists with inadvertent substitution. Milk sickness results from consumption of tremetol-contaminated milk products after fresh richweed is eaten by cattle.

Toxicity Signs/Symptoms:

Vomiting, diarrhea 6-7 hours after ingestion along with profuse sweating.

Treatment:

>   **First Aid** – Activated charcoal.

>   **Medical** – Maintain fluid and electrolyte balance; avoid the use of drugs.

References:

>   3, 5, 6, 9, 14, 101

Euphorbia corollata L.; *Euphorbia* spp.   Euphorbiaceae

Common Names:

>   Large flowering spurge, blooming spurge, milk purslane, snake milk; spurge

Parts Containing Toxins:

>   Root bark; whole plant.

>   **Toxic Constituents** – Resin.

Doses:

>   **Therapeutic** – *E. corollata* powder 65-650 mg; tincture 5-20 drops ((0.31-1.23 ml); fluid extract 1-15 drops (0.06-0.93 ml).

Note:

>   **Precautions** – Individual sensitivity may cause some patients to overreact to therapeutic doses.

>   **Contraindications** – Do not use where there is active inflammation.

>   **Mechanism of Toxicity** – The resin in the milky latex is irritating to the mucosa.

Toxicity Signs/Symptoms:

>   **Internal** – Emesis, catharsis, gastroenteritis; severe irritation of the mouth, throat and stomach.

>   **External** – Dermatitis

Treatment:

(See Treatment section under Explanation of Format.)

References:

3, 6, 8, 9, 10, 103, 104

G

Garcinia hanburyi Hooker fil.   Guttiferae

Common Names:

Gamboge, camboge, gutta gamba, tom rong

Parts Containing Toxins:

Bark exudate.

Toxic Constituents – 65-75% Gambogic acid, morellic acid, isomorellic acid (resins).

Doses:

Therapeutic – 65-194 mg (usual 125 mg).

Toxic – Gum-resin 0.2 gm.

Lethal – Gum-resin 4 gm.

Note:

Precaution – Never use alone; full doses should never be given.

Toxicity Signs/Symptoms:

Nausea and vomiting, griping, gastroenteritis, death.

Treatment:

(See Treatment section under Explanation of Format.)

Other – Alkalies.

References:

6, 7, 9, 107

Gelsemium sempervirens (L.) Aiton   Loganiaceae

Common Names:

Yellow jasmine, yellow jessamine, Carolina jasmine, woodbine

Parts Containing Toxins:

Fresh rhizome with roots; whole herb; flower nectar.

Toxic Constituents – Gelsamine, gelsemoidine, gelsemicine and sempervirine (indole alkaloids), gelseminic acid (hydroxycoumarin).

Doses:

Therapeutic – Tincture 5-30 drops (0.31-1.85 ml); fluid extract 1/2-10 drops (0.03-0.62 ml); gelsemine 0.4-1.3 mg.

Toxic – Powder 0.5 gm in child, 2-3 gm in adults.

Note:

Contraindications – In pregnancy, due to its uterine stimulant in animals, and in hypotension and respiratory or cardiac insufficiency.

Mechanims of Toxicity – Acting similar to nicotine and coniine, it first stimulates, then depresses neural function, especially in the medulla oblongata, anterior cornus of spinal cord, and spinal ganglia.

Other – The rhizome is the part used medicinally.

Symptoms may begin immediately or within one half hour.

Toxicity Signs/Symptoms:

Internal stabismus with double vision and drooping eyelids and lower jaw, dilated pupils; langor, relaxation, muscular weakness and prostration, tremors of limbs; inability to move tongue or swallow, dry mouth, loss of speech; vomiting, trembling, convulsions, sweating, skin cold and clammy; respiration slow, feeble, shallow, irregular and labored; headache, dizziness, mydriasis, amblyopia, exophthalmos; diminished rate and force of pulse, fall in temperature and blood pressure; drowsiness but easily aroused; loss of sensations; intense abdominal cramps, paralysis; cyanosis, dyspnea, consciousness preserved except in fatal doses; death from respiratory failure and cardiac embarrassment after one to seven and a half hours.

Treatment:

First Aid – Artificial respiration, emesis, charcoal, strong tea.

Medical – Gastric lavage with potassium permanganate if no emesis; castor oil purge; morphine is considered to be the best antagonist; atropine (2 mg. subcut) every four hours; mechanical ventilation with oxygen if necessary; digitalis to sustain heart action; IV diazepam for seizures; sodium bicarbonate for acidosis.

Other – Strong coffee, aromatics; external heat; nux vomica in small doses given often (every two hours); spirit of ammonia.

References:

1, 2, 3, 6, 7, 9, 10, 12, 14, 25, 103,104, 106, 107

Gentiana lutea L.   Gentianaceae

Common Names:

Gentian, bitter root, bitterwort, pale gentian, yellow gentian

Parts Containing Toxins:

Root and rhizomes (more potent fresh).

Toxic Constituents – Amarogentin, gentiopicrin, swertiamarin, sweroside (iridoid monoterpenes).

Doses:

Therapeutic – Powder 0.65-1.94 gm (usually 1 gm); fluid extract 5-30 drops (0.31-1.85 ml).

Note:

Contraindications – In acute gastro-intestinal inflammation or irritation, gastric or duodenal peptic ulcer.

Toxicity Signs/Symptoms:

Nausea, vomiting, diarrhea, fullness of pulse, headache.

Treatment:

First Aid – Emesis; activated charcoal.

Medical – Gastric lavage if no emesis; saline cathartic; maintain fluid and electrolyte balance.

References:

3, 9, 10, 14, 106, 107

Glycyrrhiza glabra L.   Fabaceae

Common Names:

Licorice, liquorice, sweet wood, sweet root

Parts Containing Toxins:

Root

Toxic Constituents – 6-14% Glycyrrhizin, also called glycyrrhizic acid or glycyrrhizinic acid (saponin glycoside).

Doses:

Therapeutic – Powder 1.0-5.0 gm (max. 5.0 gm daily); fluid extract 1-4 tsp (3.7-14.8 ml); glycyrhhizin 100 mg/day max.

Toxic – Powder more than 20 gm per day.

Note:

Precaution – Should not be used for more than 4-6 weeks without interuption.

Contraindications – In pregnancy since emmenagogue action may cause abortion. Avoid using for prolonged periods or in high doses or when pre-existent hypertension, hypokalemia, or cardiovascular disease conditions present; in diabetes, liver disorders such as cholestasis, chronic hepatitis or cirrhosis, obesity, and severe kidney insuffficiency.

Kinetics – Peak serum concentration of glycyrrhizin occurs in less than 4 hours and rapidly decreases. No glycyrrhizin is detectable after 96 hours. Up to 60% is converted by intestinal hydrolysis to the aglycone, glycyrrhetinic acid, which reaches its serum peak 24 hours after consumption of the root extract. It then gradually decreases over the next 72 hours. Most metabolites are excreted via the intestinal route.

Mechanism of Toxicity – Chronic glycyrrhetinic acid exposure inhibits 5β-reductase corticosteroid breakdown in liver, and its metabolite 3-monoglucuronyl-glycyrrhetinic acid inhibits renal 11β-hydroxysteroid dehydrogenase breakdown of cortisol, allowing it to exert mineralcorticoid effects. Glycyrrhizin and/or its metabolites also mimics aldosteronism by binding mineralcorticoid receptors and causing sodium resorption and potassium excretion by the kidneys. Myopathy appears to be due to associated with hypokalemia or hypochloremia.

Other – Chinese licorice, *Glycyrrhiza uralensis*, has equivalent components, effects, and contraindications.

Enhances corticosteroid effects when administered together including hypokalemia, high blood pressure, and edema.

Potassium depletion, especially when exacerbated by laxatives or thiazide diuretics, will increase sensitivity to cardiac glycosides.

Deglycyrrhizinated licorice is not associated with adverse side effects.

Toxicity Signs/Symptoms:

Chronic – Severe hypertension, headache, lethargy, weakness, flaccid tetraparesis, muscle pain, peripheral dysesthesia with numbness; pulmonary edema, shortness of breath, edema, weight gain; tetany, cardiac arrhythmias, heart enlargement, congestive heart failure, cardiac arrest.

Lab – Hypernatremia, hypokalemiic alkalosis; myoglobinuria; suppressed urinary aldosterone and plasma renin activity levels.

ECG – T wave changes.

Treatment:

Medical – Monitor serum potassium and sodium levels; sodium restriction; spironolactone.

Other – Eliminate licorice intake.

References:

2, 5, 14, 15, 16, 25, 60, 100, 101, 102, 106, 107, 150, 151, 152, 153, 154, 155, 156, 157, 158

H

Hedeoma pulegioides (L.) Pers.;
Mentha pulegium L.   **Lamiaceae**

Common Names:

Pennyroyal; European pennyroyal

Parts Containing Toxins:

Leaves and tops.

Toxic Constituents – Pulegone (volatile ketone) 60-80% in *H. pulegioides* and 55-95% in *M. pulegium* volatile oils.

Doses:

Therapeutic – Powder 0.32-3.24 gm; tincture 1/2-1 teaspoon (1.85-3.7 ml); oil 2-10 drops (0.12-0.62 ml).

Toxic – Oil 4-15 ml; tea 90-120 ml in infants.

Lethal – Oil 15-30 ml. LD_{50} 0.4 gm/kg orally in rats.

Note:

Precautions – Avoid oral use in liver disease or alcoholism and during use of acetominophen.

Contraindications – In pregnancy due to its emmenagogue and abortifacient effects secondary to hepatotoxicity. Do not use in pre-existing kidney disease.

Kinetics – Pulegone depletes hepatic glutathione which increases hepatotoxicity caused by pulegone. Pulegone is oxidized by hepatic cytochrome P450 system to 50% menthofuran along with other toxic metabolites. Menthofuran causes hepatic, renal, and pulmonary cellular damage. When injected IP, pulegone has a peak plasma level in 15 minutes and a half-life of 1 hour. Menthofuran peak plasma levels occurs 1 hour after IP injection of pulegone; menthofuran half-life is about 2 hours.

Gastrointestinal and central nervous system effects develop with 1-2 hours after ingestion.

Mechanism of Toxicity – Direct hepatotoxicity is caused by pulegone and its metabolic intermediates, epoxides and furans. Excretion of the oil irritates kidneys and bladder and reflexively excites uterine contraction.

Toxicity Signs/Symptoms:

Headache, dizziness, dysphagia, nausea, vomiting, diarrhea with blood, abdominal pain and cramps, dyspnea; hypertension, rash, tingling and numbness of the extremities, generalized neuromuscular atony, lethargy; gastrointestinal bleeding, constipation; shock, hematuria, vaginal bleeding; fever, delirium, twitching, seizures, convulsions, pulmonary congestion, coma and death through respiratory failure.

Fulminant hepatic failure, acute renal failure, and/or disseminated intravascular coagulation account for the most serious symptoms.

Cerebral edema, kidney damage, and hepatic necrosis have been noted on autopsy.

Lab – Elevated liver enzymes, abnormal renal function tests, metabolic acidosis, hemolytic anemia, coagulopathies, hypoglycemia.

External – Dermatitis.

Treatment:

First Aid – Emesis (Gastric lavage is preferred over ipecac if readily available due to rapid absorption of pennyroyal oil, risk of aspiration pneumonitis, and rapid onset of CNS effects.); activated charcoal (1 gm/kg body weight).

Medical – Gastric lavage if no emesis; sorbitol (2 ml/kg); cathartic.

Other – After the charcoal and sorbitol, N-acetylcysteine (190 mg/kg PO, then 70 mg/kg every 4 hours) should be given to help prevent hepatotoxicity in exposures of over 10 ml pennyroyal oil. Antioxidants such as glutathione surrogates may also be beneficial.

References:

3, 5, 6, 9, 11, 14, 17, 25, 100, 104, 105, 107, 159, 160

Helleborus niger L.   **Ranunculaceae**

Common Names:

Christmas rose, black hellebore, melampode

Parts Containing Toxins:

Roots; leaves.

Toxic Constituents – Helloborin and veratrin (steroidal saponins), hellebrin or helleborcin (steroid glycoside); helleborein (alkaloid).

Doses:

Therapeutic – Root powder 50-200 mg; tincture 2-8 drops (0.12-0.49 ml).

Note:

Contraindications – In pregnancy, especially in the first trimester, due to the use of its root as an emmenagogue and abortifacient.

Mechanism of Toxicity – Helloborin is purgative due to its irritation of the mucosa, helleborein is a narcotic, and hellebrin is a cardiac stimulant.

Other – The root is the part used medicinally.

Toxicity Signs/Symptoms:

Internal – Scratchiness in mouth and throat, salivation, GI irritation, anorexia, nausea, vomiting and diarrhea; dizziness, shortness of breath, exhaustion, spasms, convulsions, delirium, rapid pulse; numbing of oral tissue, abdominal pain, nervous effects, weakness; also, death from respiratory failure or cardiac arrest.

External – The leaves and fresh root can produce irritation of the skin.

Treatment:

First Aid – Emesis; activated charcoal; tannins and stimulants (tea or coffee). For contact dermatitis, wash twice with soap and water.

Medical – Gastric lavage; saline cathartic; catheterize to speed elimination; tincture of opium to quiet bowels; diazepam for spasms, sodium bicarbonate for acidosis; monitor and balance electrolytes; mechanical ventilation with oxygen if necessary.

Other – Keep warm.

References:

1, 3, 6, 7, 9, 10, 12, 25, 103, 104, 107

Heuchera micrantha Douglas ex Lindl.

Saxifragaceae

Common Names:

Alum root, American sanical

Parts Containing Toxins:

Root.

Toxic Constituents – 9-20% tannins.

Doses:

Toxic – Powder > 10 grams.

Note:

Kinetics – Tannins are converted to gallic acid and glucose In the intestine. Gallic acid is absorbed, degraded, and excreted in the urine.

Mechanism of Toxicity – Tannins are protein precipitants and astringents.

Other – Identified in reference 14 as nontoxic.

Toxicity Signs/Symptoms:

Gastric and renal irritation.

Treatment:

First Aid – Emesis; activated charcoal.

Medical – Gastric lavage if no emesis; saline cathartic; obtain baseline hepatic function studies.

References:

5, 14, 100

Hydrangea arborescens L.   Hydrangeaceae

Common Names:

Seven barks, wild hydrangea

Parts Containing Toxins:

Leaves, flowers and buds; branches; root.

Toxic Constituents – Hydrangin (cyanogenic glycoside).

Doses:

Therapeutic – Powdered root 2.0 gm.

Note:

The bark of the root is the part used medicinally.

Toxicity Signs/Symptoms:

Gastroenteritis and cyanide symptoms (see *Prunus* spp.); dizziness, oppressed feeling of the chest, nausea and vomiting; diarrhea with blood; rapid breathing, gasping, nervous excitement, staggering, convulsions, death.

Treatment:

First Aid – Emesis; activated charcoal.

Medical – Gastric lavage; saline cathartic; maintain fluid and electrolyte balance; amyl nitrite under nose 30 seconds each minute; IV sodium nitrite, then sodium thiosulfate; IV diazepam for seizures; emergency exchange transfusion for methemoglobulinemia.

References:

1, 5, 6, 12, 14, 100, 107

Hydrastis canadensis L.   **Ranunculaceae**

Common Names:

Goldenseal, yellow puccoon, orange root, eye balm, eye root, ground raspberry, Indian plant, jaundice root, yellow root

Parts Containing Toxins:

Root and rhizome.

Toxic Constituents – 1-3% Hydrastine, canadine (isoquinoline alkaloids), 3-4% berberine (protoberberine alkaloid).

Doses:

Therapeutic – Powder 194-972 mg; tincture 20 drops – 2 tsp (1.23-7.4 ml); Hydrastine HCl 11 mg; berberine 65-325 mg.

Toxic – Berberine sulphate 25-50 mg/kg orally in cats. (No histopathological changes were found when 0.5 gm/kg berberine sulphate daily was given orally to rats for 6 weeks.)

Lethal – Hydrastine LD_{50} 104 mg/kg IP in rats. Berberine LD_{50} 14.5 mg/kg IV, 88.5 mg/kg IP, and >1 gm/kg orally in rats; 100 mg/kg orally in cats.

Note:

Contraindications – In pregnancy due its emmenagogue effects and to uterine stimulation created in animals by its constituents berberine, hydrastine, canadine and hydrastinine.

Mechanism of Toxicity – Hydrastine is a central nervous system stimulant and has direct myocardial and intestinal smooth muscle depressant effect. Berberine depresses the myocardium in high doses and also depresses respiration, stimulates intestinal smooth muscle and reduces bronchial constriction. Canadine acts like berberine by indirectly enhancing cholinergic contractions of the intestines.

Toxicity Signs/Symptoms:

Acute – Irritation of the mouth and throat, nausea, vomiting, diarrhea, difficulty breathing, slow heart rate, spasms, paresthesia, central paralysis.

Chronic – Digestive disorder, constipation, excitation, delerium, hallucinations.

Treatment:

First Aid – Emesis; activated charcoal.

Medical – Gastric lavage with potassium permanganate if no emesis; saline cathartic; maintain fluid and electrolyte balance; sodium bicarbonate for acidosis; plasma extenders for shock; mechanical ventilation with oxygen if required; avoid the use of drugs. If necessary, use IV diazepam for spasms.

Other – Keep warm and quiet.

References:

5, 6, 9, 10, 14, 25, 49, 50, 51, 52, 100, 107

Hyoscyamus niger L.   **Solanaceae**

Common Names:

Henbane, hog's bean, Jupiter's bean, cassilata, symphonica

Parts Containing Toxins:

Whole plant.

Toxic Constituents – Scopolamine also called hyoscine, hyoscyamine, butyrine (tropane alkaloids 0.05-0.28%); hyospicrin (glucoside).

Doses:

Therapeutic – Powder 130-325 mg; tincture 2-5 drops (0.12-0.31 ml); fluid extract 1-3 drops (0.06-0.18 ml); hyoscine hydrobromate 0.33-0.93 mg.

Note:

Contraindications – Tachycardias, prostatic hyperplasia, narrow-angle glaucoma, acute pulmonary edema, stenosis of gastrointestinal tract, megacolon.

Kinetics – Decreased GI motility delays absorption.

Mechanism of Toxicity – Parasympatholytic by competitive antagonism with acetylcholine at muscarinic nerve endings, but it shows little effect on blood vessels. Activity from scopolamine is produced more strongly on iris, secretory glands and the central nervous system.

Other – Predominance of scopolamine distinguishes this plant from *Atropa belladonna* or *Datura stramonium* toxicities by causing greater central nervous system effects such as depression and then excitation.

Enhances anticholinergic action of tricyclic antidepressants, amantadine, antihistamines, phenothiazines, procainamide, and quinidine.

The leaves are the part used medicinally.

Due to its reputation as an intoxicant, this herb is subject to abuse.

Toxicity Signs/Symptoms:

Acute – Skin redness, facial dryness, dry mouth, increased pulse rate, dilated pupils, indistinct vision; nausea, vertigo, dull headache, faintness, sleepiness, muscular weakness; reduced peristalsis, constipation, elevated termperature, paralysis, giddiness, spasms, cramps, convulsions, rapid pulse, difficult urination; restlessness, mania, delirium and hallucinations, coma, and death due to asphyxiation.

Chronic – Macular rash that is dry and itching.

Treatment:

First Aid – Charcoal.

Medical – Gastric lavage with dilute Lugol's solution or potassium permanganate; saline cathartic; physostigmine IV 0.5-2 mg in 2 min; alkalize blood to pH 7.5 for arrhythmias; propanolol for tachyarrhythmias; diazepam for convulsions; chlorpromazine for severe excitation; pilocarpine hydrochloride 1/4 grain IM for peripheral neurologic deficits; mechanical ventilation with oxygen if necessary.

Other – Caffeine as supportive; sedation with brandy or tincture of opium to control delirium; lower temperature with wet cloths, not antipyretics.

References:

3, 5, 7, 8, 9, 10, 12, 13, 14, 103, 104, 106, 107

I

Inula helenium L.   Asteraceae

Common Names:

Elecampane, scabwort, alant, horseheal, yellow starwort, elfdock, elfwort, velvet dock

Parts Containing Toxins:

Roots, rhizome.

Toxic Constituents – Alantolactone and others in mixture known as helenalin (sesquiterpene lactones)

Doses:

Therapeutic – Tincture 0.5-1.0 tsp (1.85-3.7 ml); fluid extract 20-40 drops (1.23-2.47 ml).

Note:

Contraindications – In pregnancy.

Mechanism of Toxicity – The lactones irritate the mucous membranes and sensitize the skin.

Toxicity Signs/Symptoms:

Internal – Vomiting, diarrhea, cramps, and symptoms of paralysis.

External – Dermatitis can occur on contact with the rhizome.

Treatment:

First Aid – Emesis, if not spontaneous; activated charcoal. For contact dermatitis, wash twice with soap and water.

Medical – Gastric lavage if no emesis; saline cathartic; trifluoropromazine for nonproductive vomiting.

References:

100, 106, 107

Ipomoea purga Hayne.
(= *Exogonium purga* (Wend.) Bentham),
Ipomoea spp.   Convolvulaceae

Common Names:

Jalap, jalapa

Parts Containing Toxins:

Roots.

Toxic Constituents – 8-12% Convolvulin (glycosidal resin).

Doses:

Therapeutic – Powder 0.3-1.2 grams; resin 130 mg; tincture 5-20 drops (0.3-1.2 ml); fluid extract 2-10 drops (0.12-0.62 ml).

Note:

Precautions – Not to be used as a continued medication. Use with care in serious cardiac conditions.

Contraindications – In pregnancy and digestive tract inflammation.

Mechanism of Toxicity – It acts as a strong irritant to the intestinal mucosa.

Other – The use of jalap is now rare, including the species *Ipomoea orizabensis*, *Ipomoea turpenthum*, and *Ipomoea operculata*.

Toxicity Signs/Symptoms:

Extreme nausea, vomiting, griping, debilitation, violent hypercatharsis with electrolyte loss, death.

Treatment:

(See Treatment section under Explanation of Format.)

Other – *Dioscorea villosa*.

References:

3, 5, 9, 10, 107

Iris versicolor L.   Iridaceae

Common Names:

Blue flag, poison flag, flag lily, liver lily, snake lily, dragon flower, dagger flower, water flag, fleur-de-lis

Parts Containing Toxins:

Roots, rhizome, bulb, leaves, all parts.

Toxic Constituents – Iridin; irisin (resin).

Doses:

Therapeutic – Root powder 1.3 gm as cathartic; tincture 10-25 drops (0.62-1.54 ml).

Toxic – Powder 2 grams, tincture 3 tsp (11.1 ml); fluid extract 1 tsp (3.7 ml).

Note:

Contraindications – In pregnancy.

Mechanism of Toxicity – The acrid resins irritate the mucous membranes, the liver, and the pancreas.

Other – The root is the portion used medicinally.

The fresh root and plant are more irritating.

Iris virginica has similar effects and should not be used in pregnancy.

Toxicity Signs/Symptoms:

Internal – Burning sensation in mouth and throat; nausea, vomiting, violent diarrhea, abdominal burning, bloody diarrhea; difficult breathing; colic and rectal heat; gastroenteritis resulting in death.

External – Dermatitis can occur on contact with the rhizome.

Treatment:

First Aid – Charcoal; emesis. For contact dermatitis, wash twice with soap and water.

Medical – Gastric lavage if no emesis; saline cathartic; maintain fluid and electrolyte balance; avoid use of drugs;

References:

1, 5, 8, 9, 12, 14, 100, 103, 104, 107

J

Juglans cinera L.   **Juglandaceae**

Common Names:

Butternut, lemon walnut, oil nut, white walnut

Parts Containing Toxins:

Bark, leaves, hulls.

Toxic Constituents – Juglandin (resin), juglandic acid.

Doses:

Therapeutic – Tincture 1-25 drops (0.06-1.54 ml).

Note:

Contraindications – In pregnancy in large doses.

Mechanism of Toxicity – The resin is irritating to the gastrointestinal tract. Contact dermatitis occurs from contact with the juice of the leaves.

Other – The bark is the portion commonly used medicinally.

Toxicity Signs/Symptoms:

Internal – Nausea, vomiting and watery catharsis.

External – Dermatitis.

Treatment:

First Aid – For contact dermatitis, remove from source of irritant; remove contaminated clothing, wash exposed surfaces twice with soap and water.

References:

3, 9, 12, 14, 100

Juniperus communis L.   Cupressaceae

Common Names:

Juniper, common juniper

Parts Containing Toxins:

Berries (cones) with up to 3.4% volatile oil.

Toxic Constituents – 40% Alpha- and 7% beta-pinene (volatile monoterpenes) and /or 6% terpinen-4-ol (volatile alcohol) in volatile oil and probably other nonvolatile components.

Doses:

Therapeutic – Berries 4 gm; fluid extract 1/2-1 tsp (1.85-3.7 ml); oil 0.06-0.3 ml.

Toxic – Terpinen-4-ol 1.85 ml/kg orally in mice.

Lethal – Oil LD_{50} 6.28 gm/kg orally in rats; terpinen-4-ol LD_{50} 0.78 and 1.5 ml/kg IM in mice and rats, respectively.

Note:

Precautions – Frequent or prolonged repetition of the therapeutic dosage may produce toxicity. External use for large wounds, acute skin disease, fevers, cardiac insufficiency or hypertonia should only be done under a physician's supervision.

Contraindications – In pregnancy, its emmenagogic action may cause an abortion. Avoid in nephritis and pyelitis. Do not use for more than 4 weeks without medical advice.

Mechanism of Toxicity – The volatile monoterpenes are irritant to the urinary mucosa.

Other – American species including *Juniperus virginiana*, *Juniperus monosperma*, and *Juniperus osteosperma* should be regarded as having effects similar to *J. communis* and should not be used in pregnancy. The leaves of all of these species are expected to be more irritant than the berries.

Juniper oil obtained from the berries is considered by some authorities to be relatively nontoxic and safe during pregnancy. They believe the toxicity and abortifacient effects are due to nonvolatile constituents.

Toxicity Signs/Symptoms:

Acute – Catharsis; urinary suppression, dysuria, pain in kidney region, convulsions.

Chronic – Nephrosis with oliguria, personality changes, convulsions.

Lab – Hematuria and albuminuria.

Treatment:

(See the Treatment section under Explanation of Format.)

References:

3, 5, 9, 25, 34, 100, 101, 105, 106, 107

Juniperus sabina L.   Cupressaceae

Common Names:

Savin, savine

Parts Containing Toxins:

Leaves, twigs, and branch tips with 3-5% volatile oil.

Toxic Constituents – Oil with sabinyl acetate (volatile terpene ester) 20-53% of volatile oil, alpha-pinene (volatile monoterpene); podophylotoxins (lignans).

Doses:

Toxic – Volatile oil 6 drops (0.3 ml).

Note:

Precautions – Avoid oral use in liver disease or alcoholism and during use of acetaminophen.

Contraindications – In pregnancy, it acts as an embryotoxic abortifacient.

Mechanism of Toxicity – The volatiles are irritant to the intestinal mucosa and the skin.

Toxicity Signs/Symptoms:

Internal – Queasiness, spasm, kidney damage, hematuria; cardiac arrhythmias, central paralysis, unconsciousness, and death.

External – Irritation, blistering, necrosis, and poisoning from transdermal absorption.

Treatment:

First Aid – Emesis, activated charcoal.

Medical – Gastric lavage if no emesis; IV diazepam for spasms, atropine for colic; monitor and replace electrolytes; sodium bicarbonate for acidosis; monitor kidney function, blood coagulation, and liver function. Intubate and administer oxygen if necessary.

References:

105, 107

K

Kalmia angustifolia L.;
Kalmia latifolia L.   **Ericaceae**

Common Names:

Sheep's laurel, lambkill, narrow-leaved laurel; mountain laurel, broad-leaved laurel, calico bush, spoonwood

Parts Containing Toxins:

Leaves, twigs, flowers, pollen all parts.

Toxic Constituents – Andromedotoxin and others (diterpene resinoids).

Doses:

Therapeutic – Leaf powder 130-972 mg; tincture 2-15 drops (0.12-0.93 ml).

Note:

Mechanism of Toxicity – The andromedan derivatives prevent closure of sodium channels in excitable cells and block conduction.

Other – American Indians were said to have drunk a decoction of the leaves to commit suicide.

Symptoms occur 6 hours after ingestion.

Toxicity Signs/Symptoms:

Salivation, lachrymation, nasal discharge, nausea, vomiting, diarrhea; burning sensation of mouth and throat, intense abdominal pains, anorexia, paresthesias, convulsions, slow pulse, low blood pressure, paralysis, incoordination; drowsiness, dizziness, headache, muscular weakness, fever, dullness of vision; temporary loss of vision, cardiac arrhythmias, difficulty breathing, depression, prostration, paralysis of the extremities; coma, respiratory failure, cardiac arrest, death.

Treatment:

First Aid – Emesis; activated charcoal; tea or coffee.

Medical – Gastric lavage with potassium permanganate if no emesis; saline cathartic; atropine 0.6 mg IV adults; for bradycardia give phenytoin or use transvenous electrical pacemaker; for hyperkalemia give Kayeralate or glucose/insulin; sodium bicarbonate for acidosis; plasma volume expanders if required; IV diazepam for spasms; mechanical ventilation with oxygen if necessary.

Other – Whiskey; keep warm and recumbent with fresh air.

References:

1, 3, 6, 7, 9, 12, 14, 103, 104, 107

L

Larrea tridentata (Sesse. & Moc. ex DC) Covill.
Zygophyllaceae

Common Names:

Chaparral, creosote bush, greasewood

Parts Containing Toxins:

Leaves.

Toxic Constituents – Nordihydroguaiaretic acid or NDGA (lignan); resin.

Doses:

Toxic – Tea 3-4 cups daily for three months; powder 1-5 capsules or tablets daily for 1.5-12 months.

Lethal – NDGA LD_{50} of 830, 4000 and 5500 mg/kg orally in guinea-pigs, mice, and rats, respectively.

Note:

Mechanism of Toxicity – Conversion of NDGA to an O-quinone form in the ileum leads after absorption to its cysticsequestration in the kidneys as it is excreted in the urine. Hepatotoxicity appears to be idiosyncratic.

Other – Considering its history of widespread internal use, only rarely have individuals shown toxic liver reactions and then only with chronic use.

The similar South American species, *Larrea divaricata,* has also had several cases of reported contact dermatitis.

Toxicity Signs/Symptoms:

Chronic – Anorexia, nausea, vomiting, upper right quadrant pain, malaise; dark urine, jaundice, pruritus, hepatomegaly.

Along with several cases of toxic hepatitis, one case of renal cystic disease with cystic renal cell carcinoma has been reported.

In rats NDGA as 0.5-1.0% of the diet led to development of

cystic reticuloendotheliosis of paracecal lymph nodes and vaculation of kidney tubular epithelium.

Lab - Elevated liver enzymes. Liver biopsy shows active hepatitis and possibly hepatic necrosis.

Externally – Contact dermatitis.

Treatment:

Other – Cease use of herb; silymarin; monitor liver enzymes.

References:

41, 42, 43, 44, 45, 71, 101, 161, 162, 163

Linum usitatissimum L.   Linaceae

Common Names:

Flax, linseed, lint bells, linen flax

Parts Containing Toxins:

Immature seed, mature leaf, all parts.

Toxic Constituents – Linatine (glutamic acid derivative) from seeds; linamarin and lotaustralin (cyanogenic glycosides) from leaves, stems, flowers, roots, and 0.1-1.5% linustatin and neolinustatin (cyanogenic glycosides) in seeds.

Doses:

Therapeutic – Mature seeds (unground) 10-15 gm 2-3 times daily, each with a tumbler of water.

Lethal – Linatine LD_{50} 2 mg IP in week-old chicks.

Note:

Precautions – If taken with too little fluid the use of large quantities can lead to intestinal obstruction.

Contraindications – In early pregnancy, its emmenagogue action may induce abortion of the fetus. Avoid internal use of seed in intestinal obstruction, esophogeal or gastrointestinal stricture, acute gastroenteritis or esophagitis.

Mechanism of Toxicity – Linatine is hydrolized to glutamic acid and l-amino-D-proline which is a vitamin B_6 antagonist. However, the amount is too low to cause pyridoxine deficiency in humans. Linamarase (an enzyme) releases cyanide from linamarin, but linamarase is deactived in normal gastric acid.

Kinetics – The amount of hydrocyanic acid normally liberated from mature flax seeds is rapidly detoxified in the liver by rhodanase. The metabolite thiocyanate is excreted in the urine.

Other – Linseed oil boiled in driers for use in paint forms metallic salts which are poisonous.

The mature seeds are the part normally used medicinally, providing estrogenic lignans and essential fatty acids. The seeds are safe when cooked or mature.

Grinding of flax seeds to a fine powder makes the cyanogenic glycosides more liable to hydrolysis and enhances the absorption of cyanide.

Elderly people commonly are subject to achlorhydria, especially those with gastrointestinal symptomology, and therefore may not adequately deactivate the enzyme linamarase.

The seeds may delay the absorption of other drugs taken simultaneously.

Toxicity Signs/Symptoms:

Leaves – Rapid and difficult breathing; gasping, staggering, paralysis, excitement and convulsions; weakness, coma and death.

Seeds – In young chicks they cause growth inhibition after prolonged use; vitamin B_6 deficiency syndrome in chicks.

Treatment:

First Aid – Activated charcoal.

Medical – For cyanide poisoning from leaves, give gastric lavage followed by saline cathartic; amyl nitrite under nose 30 seconds each minute; sodium nitrite, then sodium thiosulfate; IV diazepam for seizures; emergency exchange transfusion for methemoglobinemia.

Other – Vitamin B_6 for long term use of seeds.

References:

2, 7, 8, 12, 14, 25, 99, 101, 102, 104, 106, 107, 111

Lobelia inflata L.   Campanulaceae

Common Names:

Indian tobacco, puke weed, emetic herb, vomitwort, asthma weed, bladderpod

Parts Containing Toxins:

Whole herb and seeds.

Toxic Constituents – Alpha-lobeline, lobelamine, and others (piperidine alkaloids 6%).

Doses:

Therapeutic – Powder 65-194 mg (usual 100 mg); tincture 5-30 drops (0.31-1.85 ml); fluid extract 1-10 drops (0.06-0.62 ml); lobeline salt 32.4-64.8 mg.

Toxic – Leaf powder 0.6-1.0 gm (some sensitive to therapeutic dose).

Lethal – Powder 4 gm.

Note:

Contraindications – In pregnancy.

Mechanism of Toxicity – Lobeline's action is similar to nicotine but 1/20-1/5 as potent. It acts as a primary stimulant and secondary depressant to preganglionic nicotinic receptors.

Other – Those who are habitual tobacco users may be less sensitive to the actions of lobeline.

Toxicity Signs/Symptoms:

Internal – Burning esophagus, salivation, nausea, vomiting, abdominal pain, burning urinary tract, anxiety, dizziness, headache, shivering, weakness, stupor, tremors, paralysis, rapid breathing, paresthesias, hypothermia, cardiac arrhythmias, rapid pulse, pinpoint pupils, unconsciousness, convulsions, coma, exhaustion, sweating, prostration, miosis, death through respiratory failure.

External – Dermatitis on contact with the leaves, stems, and fruit.

ECG – Extrasystole, sinus arrhythmia and bundle branch block.

Treatment:

First Aid – Emesis if needed; activated charcoal, tannins; coffee or tea; wash, if dermatitis.

Medical – Gastric lavage if no emesis; if early, lavage with a liter of potassium permanganate diluted 1:10,000; saline cathartic; artificial respiration; atropine 2 mg SC; opium for nervousness and pain; IV diazepam for seizures, chloral hydrate rectally for children; dopamine or phenylephrine for hypotension; monitor ECG; cardiac massage and artificial respiration may be required.

Other – Keep warm and quiet.

References:

1, 3, 4, 5, 6, 9, 10, 12, 14, 100, 107

M

Melilotus officinalis (L.) Pallas.   Fabaceae

Common Names:

Yellow sweet clover, yellow melilot, field melilot, hay flowers, king's clover

Parts Containing Toxins:

Whole herb.

Toxic Constituents – 0.4-0.9% Coumarin and melilotin, also called 3,4-dihydrocoumarin, can be transformed to bishydroxycoumarin, or dicoumarol, by the effects of frost, dry weather or mold from inadequate drying.

Doses:

Therapeutic – Powder 65-3900 mg; tincture 1-5 drops (0.06-0.3 ml).

Note:

Precautions – Avoid using in combination with salicylates.

Mechanism of Toxicity – The potential bishydroxycoumarin content may produce prolonged prothrombin and coagulation time.

Toxicity Signs/Symptoms:

Hemorrhagic diathesis internally and externally; pockets of blood swell under skin; strong heartbeat with normal or subnormal temperature. Headaches, stupor, and temporary

liver damage occur rarely in certain susceptible individuals.

Treatment:

(See Treatment section in Explanation of Format.)

References:

2, 3, 6, 8, 107

Myristica fragrans Houtt.   **Myristicaceae**

Common Names:

Nutmeg

Parts Containing Toxins:

Seeds.

Toxic Constituents – Myristicin (nonnitrogenous phenylpropenene), elemicine and safrole volatile (phenolic ether).

Doses:

Therapeutic – Powder 324-972 mg; fluid extract 10-20 drops (0.62-1.23 ml).

Toxic – Seed 1 whole ground; powder 5-15 grams;

oil > 1 ml/day of West Indian chemotype.

Lethal – Powder in excess of 12 gm; LD_{50} 2.6-6.0 gm/kg orally.

Note:

Precautions – Oral consumption of the oil should not be combined with meperidine (pethidine).

Contraindications – In pregnancy nutmeg is potentially abortifacient. The East Indian oil should not be consumed orally.

Mechanism of Toxicity – Myristicin is mildly inhibiting to monoamine oxidase.

Other – Safrole in the oil is mutagenic and carcinogenic, but no mutagenic effects have been shown for nutmeg essential oil.

Allergic contact dermatitis may occur.

The East Indian nutmeg oil chemotype is much higher in myristicin (3.3-14%) and safrole (0.6-3.3%), the two main toxic components, than West Indian nutmeg oil chemotype (0.5-0.9 % and 0.1-0.2%, respectively).

Toxicity Signs/Symptoms:

In 3-6 hours – Flushing, dry mouth, constricted pupils,

agitation, thirst, flushed face, dizziness, rapid pulse, nausea, vomiting, decreased temperature.

In 6-12 hours – Hallucinations, delirium, convulsions, neuromuscular and circulatory depression with violent headaches, drowsiness, sense of coldness, feeling of impending doom, collapse, tachycardia, feeble pulse, difficult urination and defecation; intoxication is followed by aching all over the body. Also, elation, light-headedness, floating sensation, stomach pain, liver pain, stupor, mydriasis, double vision, anxiety, panic; narcosis, collapse, coma, and death.

Treatment:

First Aid – Eemesis; activated charcoal.

Medical – Gastric lavage with potassium permanganate if no emesis; saline cathartic; physostigmine 0.5-2 mg IV; IV diazepam for spasms; atropine for colic; propanolol for tachyarrhythmias after alkalizing blood to pH 7.5; sodium bicarbonate for acidois; plasma volume expanders for shock; mechanical ventilation with oxygen if necessary.

Other – Monitor kidney function.

References:

1, 3, 4, 5, 6, 7, 9, 13, 14, 25, 100, 105, 106, 107

N

Nerium oleander L.   Apocynaceae

Common Names:

Oleander

Parts Containing Toxins:

All parts - root, leaves, flowers, and fruit.

Toxic Constituents – Oleandrin, other oleandrosides, and nerioside (steroid glycosides) and about two dozen other cardenolides.

Doses:

No ranges given.

Note:

Kinetics – Between 65-86% of the cardioactive glycosides are absorbed, and about 50% are protein bound. The duration of their effect is about 2.65 days. They are excreted through the kidneys and liver and in the milk.

Mechanism of Toxicity – Oleandrin is a derivative of gitoxigenin and acts similarly to the *Digitalis* spp. glycosides. It is positively inotropic and negatively chronotropic.

Other – It is estimated that one fourth to one third of hospital admissions from plant poisoning in Australia are due to oleander.

Poisoning may occur through inhalation of smoke from burning branches and leaves.

Toxicity Signs/Symptoms:

Nausea, vomiting, diarrhea, severe weakness, bradycardia, arrhythmias, hypotension, delierium, seizures, coma, death.

ECG – AV block with short QRS.

Lab – Hyperkalemia.

Treatment:

First Aid – Emesis in small children, activated charcoal.

Medical – Atropine and propranalol; digoxin-specific Fab antibody fragments (Digibind®).

References:

7, 93, 106, 167, 168, 169, 215, 216

Nicotiana rustica L., *Nicotiana tabacum* L.
Solanaceae

Common Names:

Tobacco

Parts Containing Toxins:

Leaves, all parts.

Toxic Constituents – Nicotine, cotinine, anabasine, nicotyrin, and others (pyridine alkaloids, 0.5-8.0%).

Doses:

Lethal – Leaf powder 2-7 gm; nicotine 40-100 mg; LD_{50} 0.58 mg/kg IV in mice.

Note:

Contraindications – Tobacco smoking should be avoided in the high risk conditions of pregnancy (mutagen and teratogen, fetotoxin, abortifacient) or while nursing, in 30-50 year old women taking birth control pills, in familial heart or vascular disease, following occupational toxin exposures, prior to surgery, and if there exists tobacco addiction or tobacco smoking-related diseases such as heart disease, ulcers, hypertension, diabetes, osteoporosis and glaucoma.

Kinetics – Nicotine is absorbed through the mucosa by respiration, orally and rectally; excreted mostly in urine, but also secreted in breast milk (0.4-0.5 mg/liter, if 10-20 cigarettes/day are smoked). Nicotine is also easily absorbed by the skin.

Mechanism of Toxicity – Causes postsynaptic stimulation of acetylcholine receptors in autonomic ganglia; in toxic doses, this is followed by prolonged blockade of transmission and depression of the effects of acetylcholine.

Other – Habituation occurs with regular use, increasing the effective and toxic doses.

Besides nicotinic effects, chronic use by smoking results in accumulation of tars and other irritants and carcinogens in the lungs.

About 11.5% of children and 15% of adults are hypersensitive to tobacco extracts with the allergen having a predilection for the vasculature. Individuals who have other allergies are more likely to have a tobacco sensitivity.

Poisoning can occur through harvesting tobacco by hand.

Toxicity Signs/Symptoms:

Acute – Nausea, dizziness, salivation, abdominal pain, vomiting, diarrhea, disturbed vision and hearing, faintness and prostration; mental confusion and marked weakness; pupils constricted and then dilated; pulse weak, slow, then rapid; blood pressure rises, then falls; respirations become irregular and convulsions appear; headaches, shaking, shivering, trembling hands, twitching, collapse; cold extremities, thirst, weakness, diminished reflexes, sweating, hyperthermia; staggering, staring, blindness, unconsciousness, cardiac arrest, death from respiratory paralysis.

Chronic – Heart disease, emphysema, chronic bronchitis, ulcers, high blood pressure, lung cancer, osteoporosis, diabetes, glaucoma, thromboembolism.

Treatment:

First Aid – Emesis if swallowed, activated charcoal.

Medical – Gastric lavage with a liter of potassium permanganate diluted 1:10,000; saline cathartic; artificial respiration with oxygen; avoid alkaline solutions; IV diazepam for seizures, chloral hydrate rectally for children; dopamine or phenylephrine for hypotension; atropine for severe sympathetic stimulation; cardiac massage; mechanical ventilation with oxygen if necessary.

Other – Do not give centrally-active analeptics.

References:

4, 6, 7, 9, 12, 13, 14, 25, 34, 107, 133, 170, 171, 172, 173

O

Oenanthe crocata L.   Apiaceae

Common Names:

Water dropwort, hemlock dropwort, dead tongue, five-fingered root, horsebane

Parts Containing Toxins:

Roots and rhizome; whole herb.

Toxic Constituents – Oenanthotoxin, oenanthetol (polyynes).

Doses:

Therapeutic – Powder 6.5-16 mg; tincture 1/20-1/4 drop (0.003-0.015 ml).

Toxic – Tincture 5 drops (0.3 ml); 1 entire root.

Note:

Mechanism of Toxicity – It causes congestion of vessels of the brain and spinal cord with serous effusion and apoplectic foci.

Other – The medicinal part is the rhizome. Plant no longer used in substance botanically only in homeopathic dilutions.

Toxicity Signs/Symptoms:

Burning in throat and stomach, nausea, gastroenteritis; violent headaches, vertigo, delirium; weakness, chills, speech disorders; tonic-clonic spasms, cardalgia, violent convulsions, sleep; loss of sight, hearing and speech, eyes roll upward; pulse slow and feeble, loss of sensory and motor powers, intellectual dullness; chills, rose-colored spots on face, breasts and arms; swollen face, bloody froth from mouth and nostrils, severe anoxia with cerebral edema resulting from the convulsions; coma, death often due to aspiration pneumonitis.

Treatment:

First Aid – CPR; emetic; keep warm, activated charcoal.

Medical – Gastric lavage with potassium permanganate if no emesis; saline cathartic; monitor cardiac function closely;

thiobarbiturates is first choice for treating spasms over IV diazepam for seizures; hemodialysis.

Other – Stimulate with brandy or ammonia.

References:

3, 6, 9, 10, 14, 103, 107

P

Papaver somniferum L.	**Papaveraceae**

Common Names:

Opium poppy, white poppy, mawseed, garden poppy

Parts Containing Toxins:

Latex from unripe seed capsules.

Toxic Constituents – Morphine, codeine, papaverine (isoquinoline alkaloids).

Doses:

Therapeutic – Powder 65-130 mg; laudanum tincture 5-20 drops (0.31-1.23 ml); codeine 15-60 mg.

Toxic – Codeine 1 mg/kg in children.

Lethal – Codeine 7-14 mg/kg in adults; 5 mg/kg in children

Note:

Contraindications – Biliary colic, acute pancreatitis; decreased respiratory reserve; pregnant or nursing mothers, children or elderly and in purulent inflammation.

Kinetics – Morphine is conjugated with glucuronic acid; codeine is metabolized by the liver, excreted in the urine. Half-life of each is 2.5-3 hours.

Mechanism of Toxicity – Morphine stimulates endorphin and enkephalin receptor sites in the central nervous system and acts as an analgesic, euphoriant, and narcotic.

Toxicity Signs/Symptoms:

Pinpoint pupils, skin clammy and pale, muscular prostration, sleep, cyanosis; nausea, vomiting, headache; constipation, pyloric spasm, intestinal atonia; respirations slow, shallow and irregular, occasional Cheyne-Stokes respiration, cyanosis; heart rate slows, blood pressure lowered, shock, insensibility, confusion; itchy skin, rashes, trembling hands, rapid pulse, dizziness; drowsiness, stupor, euphoria, delirium, coma profound; oliguria, lowered body temperature, skeletal muscles flaccid, pulmonary and brain edema; dilated pupils and sweating precede death from respiratory depression.

Treatment:

First Aid – Establish respiration; activated charcoal, strong tea and strong coffee copiously by mouth and rectum; (emesis difficult if not impossible).

Medical – Naloxone 0.4 mg is given IV as antidote, then repeated twice after 2-3 minute intervals; gastric lavage repeatedly with potassium permanganate 3-5 grains in 8 oz. water; saline cathartic; catheterize; stimulate heart with atropine hypodermically; electrolyte substitution, plasma volume expanders, treat acidosis with sodium bicarbonate; mechanical ventilation with oxygen if necessary.

Other – Rectal injection of capsicum to arouse from stupor; coffee; keep patient awake and moving; thujone; nux vomica.

References:

4, 9, 10, 12, 13, 14, 25, 103, 107

Pausinystalia yohimbe (K. Schum.) Pierre ex Beille.
(= *Corynanthe yohimbi* K. Schum.)
Rubiaceae

Common Names:

Yohimbe, johimbe

Parts Containing Toxins: Bark.

Toxic Constituents – 1.1-2.2% Yohimbine, 0.4% rauwolscine, 0.1% raubasine, alloyohimbine, corynanthine and others (indole alkaloids) 2.7-5.9% total dry bark weight.

Doses:

Therapeutic – Yohimbine HCl 2.5-6.0 mg up to three times per day.

Toxic – Yohimbine 15-60 mg orally; 0.8 mg/kg orally, 0.5 mg/kg IV. Raubasine 10-20 mg IV. Yohimbine 20 mg/kg IP or SC in mice.

Lethal – Yohimbine 300-400 mg orally in 2.5-year-old. Yohimbine LD_{50} 40 mg/kg IP or SC in mice, 0.017 mg/kg IV in mice. Raubasine LD_{50} 0.04 mg/kg IV in mice. Corynanthine LD_{50} 0.08 mg/kg IV and 185 mg/kg IP in mice.

Note:

Precaution –Yohimbine shows enhance activity in subjects with pre-existing hypertension, agoraphobia, and panic attacks.

Contraindications – In pregnancy and for children. Also avoid in angina pectoris, cardiac, liver and kidney disease, hypertension, and depression.

Kinetics – Following oral ingestion of yohimbine maximal effects are between 1-2 hours and last for 3-4 hours.

Mechanism of Toxicity – Yohimbine acts as an $alpha_2$-adrenergic antagonist.

Other – Yohimbine is more toxic than the other alkaloids in this plant.

Toxicity of yohimbine is increased by tricyclic antidepressants,

CNS stimulants, adrenergic antagonists, MOA inhibitors, and phenothiazines.

The following symptoms are indicative of oral yohimbine toxicity; they would likely be modified if the entire bark or bark extract were taken in excess.

Toxicity Signs/Symptoms:

Nausea, vomiting, hypertension, abdominal distress, salivation, mydriasis,weakness, fatigue, paralysis, loss of coordination, nervous excitation, dizziness, anxiety, panic, insomnia, severe headaches, sweating, diuresis, increased heart rate, palpitations, tachypnea, increased motor activity, irritability, bronchospasm, tremor and respiratory paralysis or cardiac failure leading to death.

Yohimbine may cause drug allergy with skin eruption, renal failure, and lupus-like syndrome.

Lab – Elevated serum catecholamines.

Treatment:

First Aid – Emesis; activated charcoal.

Medical – Gastric lavage with potassium permanganate if no emesis; saline cathartic; clonidine 0.1-0.2 mg orally for adolescents and adults; atropine; benzodiazepines for anxiety, but avoid phenothiazines; phenytoin; lidocaine or orciprenaline for cardiac rhythm disorders; transvenous electrical pacer; monitor and treat serum potassium imbalance; Kayeralate (R) or glucose/insulin for hyperkalemia; sodium bicarbonate for acidosis; plasma volume expanders for shock.

References:

5, 13, 14, 54, 55, 102, 106, 107, 175

Physostigma venenosum Balf.   Fabaceae

Common Names:

Calabar bean, ordeal bean, chop nut

Parts Containing Toxins:

Bean (seeds).

Toxic Constituents – Physostigmine (indole alkaloid).

Doses:

Therapeutic – Powder 65-194 mg; tincture 3-10 drops (0.18-
0.62 ml); physostigmine sulfate or salicylate 0.43-2.16 mg.

Lethal – Physostigmine 6-10 mg.

Note:

Contraindications – Asthma, gangrene, cardiovascular disease or
mechanical obstruction of GI or GU tract.

Mechanism of Toxicity – Physostigmine acts as a
parasympathomimetic due to its anticholinesterase activity in
reducing the breakdown of acetylcholine.

Toxicity Signs/Symptoms:

Dizziness, faintness, nausea, vomiting, diarrhea, salivation,
pinpoint pupils, dysphagia, dyspnea, prostration; sweating,
lacrimation, tremor, muscular weakness, respiratory depression;
peristalsis with involuntary defecation and urination; cold
extremities, hypotension, slow, feeble or irregular pulse;
bronchial constriction, wheezing, cyanosis; paralysis, twitching
muscles, fainting, convulsions; paralysis, laryngospasm. CNS
effects include confusion, ataxia, slurred speech, loss of reflexes,
coma; death due to respiratory failure.

Treatment:

Medical – Gastric lavage with 0.2% potassium permanganate;
atropine 2 mg IM every 3-10 minutes until the pulse quickens,
then orally, if necessary. Pralidoxine as cholinesterase reactivator;
trimethadone for convulsions; diazepam for spasms. Forced
diuresis; mechanical ventilation with oxygen if necessary.

Other – Nux vomica may be used as a supportive aid, or coffee or tea. External heat; treat shock.

References:

3, 6, 9, 10, 13, 14, 103, 107

Phytolacca americana L. (= *Phytolacca decandra* L.)   Phytolaccaceae

Common Names:

Poke, pokeweed, garget, inkberry, pigeon berry, scoke, red weed

Parts Containing Toxins:

All; potency diminishes from root to stems, leaves, to green fruit.

Toxic Constituents – Phytolaccatoxin, phytolaccosides (triterpene saponins), mitogens (proteins) and resin.

Doses:

Therapeutic – Powdered root 65-1300 mg; tincture 1-30 drops (0.06-1.85 ml).

Toxic – Powdered root > 1.95 gm.

Lethal – Berries or root 0.5 ounce (15.55 gm); 10 berries in infants. Saponin LD_{50} 0.065 mg/kg IP in mice.

Note:

Contraindications – In pregnancy since it acts as a uterine stimulant in animals and is possibly abortifacient.

Mechanism of Toxicity – The saponins are irritants, causing emesis and catharsis.

Other – Fresh plant material is the most potent.

Toxicity increase with plant maturity, except the reverse is true for the berries.

Toxicity reduced by heating plant substance.

Inhalation of the root powder leads to respiratory irritation and gastroenteritis. Symptoms come after 2 hours.

Toxicity Signs/Symptoms:

Burning in mouth, throat, and stomach, nausea, persistent vomiting and watery or bloody diarrhea from gastroenteritis, severe abdominal cramps, ulcerative gastritis; slowed respiration, drowsiness, prickling and tingling over entire body, weakness, profuse sweating, vertigo, cold skin, prostration; slows heart and pulse, reduced blood pressure, depression of visual and auditory senses, drowsiness, amblyopia; severe thirst, salivation, headache, dizziness; then, dyspnea, gross tremors of the hands, tachycardia, incontinence, confusion, lethargy, stupor, tetanic convulsions; recovery occurs after 24 hours, or, coma and death by respiratory paralysis.

Lab – Plasmacytosis of peripheral blood with both mature and immature cell forms which may persist for 2 or more months.

Treatment:

First Aid – Emetic; activated charcoal.

Medical – Gastric lavage with potassium permanganate if no emesis; opiates to relieve irritation; saline cathartic; IV diazepam for seizures; sodium bicarbonate for acidosis.

Other – Brandy or ammonia; demulcents and observe vital signs for supportive care.

References:

1, 3, 5, 6, 7, 8, 9, 10, 12, 14, 25, 61, 101, 107, 178

Picrasma excelsa (Swartz) Planch.

Simaroubaceae

Common Names:

Quassia, Jamaican quassia, bitter wood

Parts Containing Toxins:

Wood of the trunk and branches.

Toxic Constituents – Quassin (triterpene glycoside).

Doses:

Therapeutic – Powder 0.65-1.94 gm; tincture 2-4 ml; fluid extract 1-2 ml.

Note:

Precautions – Established doses should not be exceeded. Toxicity may occur in children even from rectal injections.

Contraindications – In pregnancy.

Mechanism of Toxicity – The bitters cause irritation of the gastric mucosa.

Other – The related plant, *Quassia amara,* has similar uses and effects and is also contraindicated in pregnancy.

Toxicity Signs/Symptoms:

Acute – Vomiting, collapse.

Chronic – Weak vision, blindness possible.

Treatment:

(See Treatment section of Explanation of Format.)

References:

3, 6, 9, 100, 103, 107

Pilocarpus jaborandi Holmes., *Pilocarpus microphyllus* Stapf.   Rutaceae

Common Names:

Jaborandi, juarandi

Parts Containing Toxins:

Dried leaflets.

Toxic Constituents – Pilocarpine (imidazole alkaloid).

Doses:

Therapeutic – Powder 1.3-3.9 gm; fluid extract 5-60 drops (0.31-3.7 ml); pilocarpine HCl 5.4-10.8 mg.

Lethal – Powder 5-10 gm; pilocarpine 60 mg.

Note:

> **Contraindications** – In pregnancy since it acts as a teratogen and as a uterine stimulant in animals. In feebleness, asthma, weak heart action, tendency to depression.

> **Mechanism of Toxicity** – Pilocarpine acts as a parasympathomimetic through stimulation at the postsynaptic neuroeffector junction.

> **Other** – *Pilocarpus pennatifolius* has similar effects and is also contraindicated in pregnancy.

Toxicity Signs/Symptoms:

> Increased flow of saliva, tears and sweat; increased thirst with nausea upon drinking water; vomiting, abdominal pains, diarrhea; miosis and blurred vision; bronchial spasm, dyspnea, convulsions, low blood pressure, vertigo, hiccough, weakness, slow heart rate, circulatory depression, palpitations, collapse, rarely death from respiratory failure or exhaustion with pre-existing cardiac disease.

Treatment:

> **Medical** – Atropine (or belladonna); gastric lavage following tannic acid or potassium permanganate; opium tincture for GI symptoms; counteract pulmonary edema.

> **Other** – Tinctures of ginger or capsicum; cardiac and respiratory support such as nux vomica, caffeine, or strophanthus given early, then followed with cactus or digitalis; strong coffee.

References:

> 3, 6, 9, 10, 13, 25, 100, 107

Piper methysticum G. Forster.   **Piperaceae**

Common Names:

> Kava, kava-kava, kawa, ava pepper, intoxicating pepper

Parts Containing Toxins:

> Root (rhizome).

Toxic Constituents – Kavain, methysticin, yongonine, and others (kavalactones 5-12%).

Doses:

Therapeutic – Root 2.0-4.0 gm as a decoction; kavalactones 60-600 mg daily.

Note:

Precautions – Do not use more than 3 months without medical advice.

Contraindications – In pregnancy and by nursing mothers and in endogenous depression.

Mechanism of Toxicity – Kava appears to have dopamine antagonistic properites.

Other – May potentiate psycholpharmacologic agents such as barbiturates and alcohol.

May adversely affect operation of motor vehicles.

Toxicity Signs/Symptoms:

Acute – Dyskinesias.

Chronic – Yellow discoloration of skin, hair and nails; accommodative disturbances, enlarged pupils, disturbed oculomotor equilibrium. Scaly skin reactions beginning at the head and moving downward.

Treatment:

Other – Cease consumption of root and its extracts.

References:

100, 106, 107, 176, 177

Piscidia erythrina L.   Fabaceae

Common Names:

Jamaica dogwood

Parts Containing Toxins:

Root bark.

Toxic Constituents – Piscidin (glycoside), rotenone.

Doses:

Therapeutic – Powder 0.33- 3.9 gm;

tincture 5-30 drops (0.3-1.8 ml).

Toxic – Fluid extract 2 ml.

Note:

Though used as a fish poison, it is non-toxic when fed to rats in massive oral doses.

Reference 14 states that *Piscidia* is not considered dangerous.

Toxicity Signs/Symptoms:

Destroys sensation; salivation, perspiration, mydriasis, diminished reflexes, nausea, vomiting, general weakness, diminished pulse force and rate, lowered blood pressure and reduced respiratory volume and rate, dyspnea, convulsions, paralysis, death from respiratory paralysis.

Treatment:

First Aid – Establish respiration; emesis; activated charcoal.

Medical – Gastric lavage if no emesis; cathartic; treat hypotension with fluids; IV diazepam for convulsions; respirator if there is CNS depression.

References:

3, 5, 9, 10, 14, 62

Podophyllum peltatum L.   Berberidaceae

Common Names:

American mandrake, duck's foot, mayapple, ground lemon, hog apple, Indian apple, raccoon berry, wild lemon

Parts Containing Toxins:

Root, rhizomes, young shoots and unripe fruit.

Toxic Constituents – 3.5-6% Podophyllin (gum resin)

containing podophyllotoxin (20%), alpha-peltatin (5%) and beta-peltatin (10%) (lignans).

Doses:

Therapeutic – Powder 325-1950 mg; tincture 1/10-10 drops (0.01-0.62 ml); resin 10 mg.

Toxic – Powdered root 2-4 gm; resin 0.3-1 gm (externally).

Lethal – Resin in elderly as little as 300-350 mg internally; LD_{50} 33 mg/kg IP in mice, 15 mg/kg IP in rats.

Note:

Precautions – Do not apply on skin surface area greater than 25 cm^2 (2.3 in. x 2.3 in.). Do not apply near eyes. Wash the site of application after 4-8 hours.

Contraindications – In pregnancy (teratogenic and feticidal); 30 mg of resin is teratogenic.

Kinetics – Absorbed orally and cutaneously; eliminated in the bile with a half-life of 48 hours.

Mechanism of Toxicity – The peltatins are the primary irritants to bowel mucosa. Podophyllotoxin and the peltatins are also growth inhibitors, by arresting cell mitosis in metaphase.

Other – Salt increases its toxicity.

The fruit is the only part that is edible.

Podophyllum hexandrum, also known as *Podophyllum emodi*, has twice as much of the toxic constituents and similar effects, so it is also contraindicated in pregnancy.

Toxicity Signs/Symptoms:

External – Dermatitis; keratitis, conjunctivitis; erythema, edema, erosion, ulceration.

Internal – Nausea, diarrhea with griping, hyperemesis, gastrointestinal ulceration, drowsiness, lethargy and unconsciousness in 12-24 hours; dizziness, poor coordination, headache, respiratory stimulation, tachycardia, hypotension, nephritis, oliguria; hallucinations, paresthesias in fingers, hands and/or feet, collapse, coma; death due to gastroenteritis or respiratory failure.

Peripheral neuropathy may not appear until weeks after application or ingestion, but it persists for months.

Lab – Leucopenia, anemia, thrombocytopenia; hypokalemia, hypocalcemia, lactic acidosis.

Treatment:

First Aid – Dilute with fluids; emesis; maintain hydration; activated charcoal. For dermatitis wash well twice with soap and water.

Medical – Gastric lavage with potassium permanganate if no emesis; saline cathartic; diazepam for spasms; Trendelenburg position and IV fluids for hypotension; platelets and whole blood; hemodialysis if renal failure; baseline CBC, electrolytes, renal and hepatic function tests; sodium bicarbonate for acidosis; plasma volume expanders for shock; mechanical ventilation with oxygen if necessary.

Other – Alkalies, aromatics, hyoscyamus or leptandra for griping; observe 6-10 hours after symptom free.

References:

1, 3, 5, 6, 7, 8, 9, 12, 14, 22, 63, 64, 65, 66, 67, 100, 101, 106, 107

Polygala senega L.   Polygalaceae

Common Names:

Seneca snakeroot, senega, rattlesnake root, milkwort, mountain flax

Parts Containing Toxins:

Root.

Toxic Constituents – 6-16% Senegasaponins A-D (triterpene saponins) with aglycone presenegenin or senegin.

Doses:

Therapeutic – Powder 0.5-1.0 gm; fluid extract 10-20 drops (0.62-1.24 ml).

Lethal – Saponins LD_{50} 3 mg/kg parenterally in rats.

Note:

Precautions – Not for long term use.

Contraindications – In pregnancy due to its uterine stimulant activity and emmenagogue effect, and in gastritis and gastric ulcers.

Mechanism of Toxicity – It acts as a skin irritant and strong gastrointestinal irritant.

Toxicity Signs/Symptoms:

Nausea and vomiting, diarrhea, CNS depression.

Treatment:

(See Treatment section in Explanation of Format.)

References:

5, 10, 25, 100, 106, 107

Polymnia uvedalia L.   Asteraceae

Common Names:

Bearsfoot, uvedalia, leaf cup

Parts Containing Toxins:

Root.

Toxic Constituents – Balsamic resin.

Doses:

Therapeutic – Powder 325-1950 mg; tincture 10-30 drops (0.62-1.85 ml).

Toxicity Signs/Symptoms:

Gastrointestinal inflammation with vomiting and diarrhea, convulsions and death.

Treatment:

(See Treatment section in Explanation of Format.)

References:

3, 9

Prunus armeniaca L.;
Prunus dulcis (Mill.) D.A. Webb var. *amara* (DC.)
    H.E. Moore.;
Prunus persica (L.) Batsch.   **Rosaceae**

Common Names:

Apricot; Bitter almond; Peach

Parts Containing Toxins:

Seeds (pits); also bark, leaves.

Toxic Constituents – In pits <8.0%, 1.0-8.0%, and 2.0-6.0% amygdalin (cyanogenic glycoside), respectively.

Concentration of toxin varies with species, climate and time of year.

Doses:

Therapeutic – Tincture of leaves 2-15 drops (0.12-0.92 ml).

Toxic – Bitter almond pits 3; apricot pits 20-40.

Lethal – Bitter almond pits 40-60 (children 7-10). Aprikern 20 capsules (child 5 capsules).

Laetril tabs 10 grams; hydrocyanic acid 50-60 mg; bitter almond oil LD_{50} 0.96 gm/kg orally in animals.

Note:

Contraindications – The seeds of *P. persica* in pregnancy due to their emmenagogue and abortifacient effects and the potential toxicity from amygdalin. The aromatic oil of bitter almond should not be used internally or externally in therapy.

Kinetics – Rhodanese in liver converts amygdalin to thiocyanate, but not rapidly enough. This is speeded by sodium thiosulfate. Intestinal flora hydrolizes amygdalin.

Mechanism of Toxicity – In crushed, moistened seeds, beta-glucosidase catalyzes hydrolysis to cyanide, speeded by alkaline pH. Hydrocyanic acid forms a stable complex with cytochrome oxidase, resulting in cellular hypoxia.

Toxicity Signs/Symptoms:

Acute – Onset in 1/2-2 hours; sudden vomiting and GI pain; rapid breathing, then respiratory depression; syncope, lethargy, coma, convulsions, death.

Chronic – Sensory and motor ataxia, optic atrophy and nerve deafness.

Treatment:

First Aid – Establish respiration; emesis; activated charcoal.

Medical – Gastric lavage, cathartic; amyl nitrite under nose 30 sec. each minute; injections of dicobalt-EDTA solution. Sodium nitrite followed by sodium thiosulfate; diazepam for seizures; emergency exchange transfusion for methemoglobinemia, not methylene blue. Mechanical ventilation may be required.

References:

5, 6, 7, 12, 14, 25, 100, 105, 107

Prunus serotina Ehrh., *Prunus virginiana* L.   **Rosaceae**

Common Names:

Wild cherry, wild black cherry, choke cherry, black cherry

Parts Containing Toxins:

Bark, seeds, leaves.

Toxic Constituents – 0.5-1.5% Prunasin & amygdalin (cyanogenic glycosides).

Doses:

Therapeutic – Powder 2.0-4.0 gm; tincture 5-30 drops (0.31-1.85 ml).

Note:

Precautions – Not for long term use; do not exceed recommended dose.

Contraindications – In pregnancy due to cyanogenic glycosides which can be teratogenic.

Mechanism of Toxicity – The glycosides in large amounts can produce cyanide poisoning, with resultant cellular hypoxia.

Other – The bark is the part used medicinally.

Prunasin is higher in bark that is actively photo-synthesizing (green).

Toxicity Signs/Symptoms:

Difficult breathing, spasms, stupor, vocal cord paralysis, twitching, convulsions, coma, death.

Treatment:

First Aid – Emesis.

Medical – Gastric lavage after antidoting with sodium nitrite IV and thiosulfate; amyl nitrate inhalation 1 ampule every 5 minutes for cyanide poisoning; artificial respiration with 100% oxygen; cathartic; IV diazepam for seizures; emergency

exchange transfusion for methemoglobulinemia; dicobalt-EDTA solution injection.

References:

1, 6, 7, 8, 12, 14, 100, 104, 107

Pulsatilla pratensis (L.) Miller
(= *Anemone pratensis* L.),
Pulsatilla vulgaris Miller
(= *Anemone pulsatilla L.)*   **Ranunculaceae**

Common Names:

Wind flower, pasque flower, passe flower, meadow anemone, Easter flower

Parts Containing Toxins:

Fresh plant; dried herb.

Toxic Constituents –Ranunculin (lactone) enzymatically converted to protoanemonin when crushed fresh.

Doses:

Therapeutic – Powder 65-324 mg; tincture 5-30 drops (0.31-1.85 ml); fluid extract 1/2-10 drops (0.03-0.62 ml).

Note:

Contraindications – In pregnancy due to its uterine stimulant activity and emmenagogue effect, as well as its teratogenic effects in animals.

Mechanism of Toxicity – Protoanemonin is a strong mucous membrane irritant, especially for the genitourinary tract.

Other – Dermitis occurs from handling the fresh plant.

Protoanemonin dimerizes to yield anemonin.

External and internal toxicity diminishes with drying.

Toxicity Signs/Symptoms:

Internal – Burning sensation in mouth and throat, salivation, colic, abdominal pain, nausea, vomiting and bloody diarrhea; urinary tract irritation, pulse slow and feeble, cardiac arrhythmia, weakness, slow and difficult respiration; mydriasis, hypothermia, sensory and motor depression or paralysis, stupor, coma and convulsions.

External – Dermatitis; vesiculation with prolonged exposure.

Treatment:

> **First Aid** – Emesis, if necessary; activated charcoal. For contact dermatitis, wash exposed area and clothing twice with soap and water.

> **Medical** – Gastric lavage with diluted potassium permanganate if no emesis.

> **Other** – Demulcents.

References:

> 3, 5, 6, 9, 10, 12, 14, 25, 103, 106, 107

Punica granatum L.   Punicaceae

Common Names:

> Pomegranate, grenadier

Parts Containing Toxins:

> Dried root bark, seeds.

> **Toxic Constituents** – Pelletrin, isopelletierin, methyl-isopelletierin, and pseudopelletierin (piperidine alkaloids 0.4%); punicalagin, punicacortein C, casuarin (tannins 20-25%).

Doses:

> **Therapeutic** – Powder 325-1800 mg; tincture 5-45 drops (0.31-2.77 ml).

> **Toxic** – Tincture 60 ml every 2-4 hours.

> **Fatal** – Powder > 80 gm.

Note:

> **Contraindications** – In pregnancy due to its emmenagogue and possible abortifacient, effects, confirmed by its uterine stimulant activity in animals.

> **Mechanism of Toxicity** – The tannins cause gastric irritation, while the alkaoids are stimulants similar to strychnine.

Toxicity Signs/Symptoms:

> Nausea, vomiting, dizziness, abdominal cramps, diarrhea; chills,

muscular incoordination, transient diplopia and amblyopia, transient blindness (occasionally permanent) after a few hours or days, mydriasis, headache, vertigo, drowsiness, collapse, respiratory failure and death.

Treatment:

First Aid – Establish respiration; emesis; activated charcoal.

Medical – Gastric lavage with potassium permanganate solution; saline cathartic; IV diazepam for spasms, sodium bicarbonate for acidosis, plasma volume expanders for shock; electrolyte substitution; mechanical ventilation with oxygen if necessary.

Other – Obtain baseline hepatic studies; monitor kidney function; keep quiet and warm.

References:

3, 5, 14, 25, 107

R

Ranunculus spp.	Ranunculaceae

Common Names:

Buttercup, crowfoot, goldcup

Parts Containing Toxins:

Whole fresh herb, except seeds (most toxic in flowering stage).

Toxic Constituents – Ranunculin (lactone) enzymatically converted to protoanemonin when crushed fresh.

Doses:

Therapeutic – Tincture 6-8 drops (0.37-0.49 ml).

Note:

Contraindications – In pregnancy due to reflex irritations. The plant contains 5-hydroxy-tryptamine which is a uterine stimulant in animals.

Mechanism of Toxicity – Protoanemonin is a strong mucous membrane irritant, especially for the gastrointestinal and genitourinary tract.

Other – The toxicity is abolished by drying or cooking.

Protoanemonin dimerizes to yield anemonin.

Toxicity Signs/Symptoms:

Internal – Gastrointestinal irritation, with vomiting and diarrhea with bleeding; burning sensation in mouth and pharynx; salivation, stomatitis, sometimes with blisters and ulceration; depression, slow pulse, dizziness, fainting, jerky spasms, convulsions, temporary blindness; polyuria, hematuria, pain, followed by oliguria due to renal damage.

External – Dermatitis, blisters..

Treatment:

First Aid – Emesis; activated charcoal. For dermatitis, wash twice with soap and water.

Medical – Gastric lavage with dilute potassium permanganate if no emesis; saline cathartic; maintain fluid and electrolyte balance; avoid use of drugs;

References:

1, 6, 7, 12, 14, 25, 103, 107

Rauvolfia serpentina (L.) Bentham ex Kurz
Apocynaceae

Common Names:

Rauwolfia, Indian snakeroot, snakewood

Parts Containing Toxins:

Root.

Toxic Constituents – Reserpine, serpentinine, raupine, ajmaline, and others (indole alkaloids)

Doses:

Therapeutic – Powder 50-300 mg; reserpine 0.1-0.25 mg.

Toxic – Reserpine 0.25-260 mg.

Lethal – Reserpine LD50 10 mg/kg IV in rabbits and rats.

Note:

Contraindications – In pregnancy since it has both teratogenic and abortifacient potential, containing the animal uterine stimulants ajmaline, coryanthine and reserpine. Also avoid if nursing or if there is a history of depression, pheochromocytoma, or peptic ulcers.

Kinetics – Half-life 11.5-16 days, independent of renal function; 6% excreted in urine the first day.

Mechanism of Toxicity – Reserpine is an antiadrenergic that depletes serotonin. Reserpine inhibits the binding of norepinephrine into the vesicles, leading to its breakdown by MAO and ultimately depletes this neurotransmitter. Its effects are both central (anti-psychotic; vasomotor center) and peripheral (antihypertensive).

Other – Diminished reaction time is exacerbated by combining its use with alcohol. It also potentiates neuroleptics and barbiturates.

It should not be combined with digitalis glycosides (bradycardia), levodopa (extra-pyramidal motor symptoms), or sympathomimetics (hypertension).

The following toxicity symptoms include those for the alkaloid reserpine.

Toxicity Signs/Symptoms:

Sedation, depression, fatigue, diminished libido, nightmares, abdominal cramps, diarrhea, intense gastric acid secretion; gastrointestinal ulceration and hemorrhage, water retention, nasal congestion; extrapyramidal disturbances and flushing of the skin; pinpoint pupils; hypotension, bradycardia and decreased temperature occur after the tachycardia; vertigo, stupor, tremors and coma. Symptoms may last from 3 hours to 7 days.

Treatment:

First Aid – Emesis or gastric lavage; activated charcoal.

Medical – Cathartic; atropine for Parkinsonism or GI hyperactivity; metaraminol or levarteranol for hypotension; avoid digitalis in cardiac failure.

Other – Use blankets for hypothermia; administer fluids for hypotension; monitor cardiac function and blood pressure closely.

References:

4, 5, 6, 7, 13, 14, 25, 106, 107

Rhamnus frangula L.
(= *Frangula alnus* Miller)   Rhamnaceae

Common Names:

Frangula, alder buckthorn, alder dogwood, arrow-wood, black alder dogwood, black alder tree, black dogwood, European black alder, European buckthorn

Parts Containing Toxins:

Dried bark.

Toxic Constituents – Emodin, chrysophanol (anthraquinones); frangulin A & C (anthraquinone glycosides).

Doses:

Therapeutic – Infuse 2.0 gm as a tea; fluid extract 1.85-3.7 ml.

Note:

Precautions – Use bark that has been dried at least one year. Do not use in excess of 8-10 days.

Contraindications – In pregnancy, nursing mothers, and in children under age 12. Also in patients with intestinal obstruction, abdominal pain of unknown origin, and any intestinal inflammation including appendicitis.

Mechanism of Toxicity – The anthranoids act as irritants to GI mucosa, stimulating propulsive contractions and chloride secretion. When the bark is used fresh, there is also an emetic action.

Other – The berries of a related species, *Rhamnus catharticus,* has similar uses and effects and is also contraindicated in pregnancy, children, and intestinal inflammation and obstruction.

The loss of potassium with prolonged use increases sensitivity to cardiac glycoside medications.

Toxicity Signs/Symptoms:

Acute – Violent vomiting and catharsis, abdominal cramping pain, collapse, dizziness, kidney damage, oliguria.

Chronic – Electrolyte loss, hyperaldosteronism, reduced intestinal motility, heart arrhythmias, nephropathies, edema, accelerated bone deterioration.

Lab – Hypokalemia, albuminuria, hematuria, proteinuria.

Treatment:

First Aid – Emesis; activated charcoal.

Medical – Gastric lavage if no emesis; maintain fluid and electrolyte balance; avoid use of drugs.

References:

3, 5, 6, 14, 100, 101, 106, 107

Rhamnus purshiana DC.   Rhamnaceae

Common Names:

Cascara sagrada, sacred bark, chittim bark, California bukthorn

Parts Containing Toxins:

Dried bark.

Toxic Constituents – Emodin, aloin (anthraquinones), cascarosides A-F (anthraquinone glycosides).

Doses:

Therapeutic – Powder 0.3-1.0 gm; fluid extract 10-60 drops (0.62-3.7 ml).

Note:

Precautions – Do not use in excessive or continuous doses (not more than 8-10 days). Do not use fresh bark (dried less than one year).

Contraindications – In pregnancy and in children under age twelve. Also in patients with intestinal obstruction, abdominal pain of unknown origin, intestinal inflammation, chronic bowel disease or ulcers.

Mechanism of Toxicity – The anthraquinones are an irritant/stimulant to intestines that increase propulsive contractions and chloride secretion.

Other – The loss of potassium with prolonged use or combined with thiazide diuretics, corticosteroids, or licorice increases sensitivity to cardiac glycoside medications.

Toxicity Signs/Symptoms:

Acute – Griping with extensive diarrhea, accompanied by nausea and vomiting, abdominal pain, kidney damage.

Chronic – Electrolyte loss, hyperaldosteronism, reduced intestinal motility, heart arrhythmias, nephropathies, edema, accelerated bone deterioration.

Lab – Hypokalemia, albuminuria, hematuria, proteinuria.

Treatment:

First Aid – Emesis; activated charcoal.

Medical – Gastric lavage if no emesis.

Other – Maintain fluid and electrolyte balance; avoid use of drugs.

References:

3, 5, 14, 100, 106, 107

Rheum officinale Baill., *Rheum palmatum* L.   Polygonaceae

Common Names:

Rhubarb, turkey rhubarb, Chinese rhubarb

Parts Containing Toxins:

Leaf blades. Root.

Toxic Constituents – Oxalic acid. Emodin, chrysophanol, aloe-emodin, rhein (anthraquinones) and their glucosides; oxalates, tannins.

Doses:

Therapeutic – Root powder 0.32-1.94 gm; tincture 5-35 drops (0.31-2.16 ml); fluid extract 5-15 drops (0.31-0.93 ml).

Toxic – 1 or more leaves.

Note:

Precautions – Not for use in excess of 8-10 days. Individual with a history of kidney stones should not use frequently.

Contraindications – In pregnancy since the roots acts as a uterine stimulant in animals. Its use should be avoided while nursing and for children under age twelve, in intestinal obstruction, if there is abdominal pain of unknown origin, and in any intestinal inflammation including appendicitis.

Mechanism of Toxicity – The anthraquinones are an irritant/stimulant to intestines stimulating propulsive contractions and chloride secretion.

Other – Only the roots and rhizomes are used medicinally. The roots of *Rheum rhaponticum* or the garden rhubarb *Rheum undulatum* contain the stilbene derivative rhaponticin with estrogen-like activity, and the leaves of these species also can cause oxalate poisoning.

Chronic use may lead to potassium deficiency with disorders of heart function and muscular weakness, especially if combined with thiazide diuretics, corticosteroids or licorice. Low potassium enhances sensitivity to cardiac glycosides.

The root of the similar species, *Rheum tanguticum,* has similar effects and the same contraindications in pregnancy, children, and intestinal obstruction and inflammation.

Toxicity Signs/Symptoms:

Leaves – Weakness, irritation in the mouth and throat; nausea, vomiting, diarrhea, abdominal pain, reduced urine formation, hemorrhages (impaired blood clotting), convulsions, salivation, headache, staggering, difficulty breathing; then, coma and death 3-5 hours after symptoms appear. It sometimes takes 1-2 days before abdominal pain begins.

Roots – Diarrhea with griping; icterus and liver enlargement, with renal insufficiency and proteinuria.

Treatment:

First Aid – [Leaves] Cold to mouth. Precipitate oxalate by giving calcium in any form orally, including milk, chalk, calcium gluconate, chloride or lactate mixed with emesis fluids. Charcoal.

Medical – [Leaves] Gastric lavage if no emesis; cathartic. Treat as for acid indigestion. IV calcium gluconate for tetany.

Other – [Leaves/Roots] Monitor BUN and creatinine. If renal function remains normal, give fluids to 4 liters daily to prevent precipitation of calcium oxalate in renal tubules.

References:

1, 3, 5, 6, 7, 8, 12, 14, 25, 100, 101, 104, 106, 107

Ricinus communis L.   Euphorbiaceae

Common Names:

Castor bean, palma Christi, Mexico seed, castor-oil plant

Parts Containing Toxins:

Seeds; leaves, young seedlings.

Toxic Constituents – 3% Ricin (toxalbumin); ricinine.

Doses:

Therapeutic – Oil 5-20 ml.

Toxic – Seeds 2-4 (adults).

Lethal – Seeds 2-4 (children); 8-12 seeds for adults; ricin LD50 0.1 ug (mice).

Note:

Precautions – Do not use oil in excess of 8-10 days or in children under age twelve.

Contraindications – In pregnancy the oil can act as a human abortifacient. It should be avoided in intestinal obstruction and abdominal pain of unknown origin.

Other – Frequent use of the oil may lead to gastric irritation or allergic skin reactions and increases potassium loss which can enhance sensitivity to cardiac glycosides.

The toxic seeds, seedlings and leaves are not used as remedies internally.

Ricin is not extracted from the seeds into the commonly used medicinal laxative oil, nor is it absorbed well from the GI tract. Ricin is one of the most toxic plant substances known.

Toxicity Signs/Symptoms:

[Oil] Gasric irritation, nausea, vomiting, colic, severe diarrhea.

[Seeds internally] Burning of mouth and throat, thirst, vomiting, stomach pain, dull weak rapid pulse, uremia; severe gastroenteritis with diarrhea, colic; 2-5 days later symptoms appear of: headache, dizziness, dullness of vision, depression, liver and kidney damage; retinal, scleral, or CNS hemorrhage; sweating, trembling, weakness; circulatory collapse, convulsions and death up to 12 days after ingestion, usually due to hypovolemic shock.

Lab – Greatly increased SGOT, SGPT, and LDH; hypoglycemia.

Treatment:

First Aid – [Seeds] Emesis; activated charcoal; keep warm and quiet.

Medical – [Seeds] Gastric lavage with potassium permanganate if no emesis; saline cathartic; IV diazepam for spasms; force fluids;

sodium bicarbonate for acidosis; electrolyte replacement; plasma volume expanders for shock; papain to hydrolyze unabsorbed lectins.

Other – [Seeds] Vitamin C; monitor fluid and electrolyte balance; alkalinize with calcium, sodium or potassium carbonate and maintain good urine flow; monitor vital signs frequently; monitor kidney function and blood coagulation.

[Leaves] For dermatitis, wash twice with soap and water.

References:

6, 7, 8, 12, 14, 25, 100, 101, 104, 107, 179

Rumex crispus L.   Polygonaceae

Common Names:

Yellow dock, curled dock, garden patience, narrow dock, sour dock

Parts Containing Toxins:

Fresh leaves. Root.

Toxic Constituents – Potassium oxalate, calcium oxalate. Chrysophanol, emodin (anthraquinones); tannins.

Doses:

Therapeutic – Powdered root 778 mg.

Toxic – 1 or more fresh leaves.

Note:

Mechanism of Toxicity – Calcium oxalate crystals in the leaves mechanically penetrate tissue, thus creating many small wounds. Anthrones in the fresh root irritate the gastrointestinal mucosa.

Other – The root is the part used medicinally.

Oxalate crystals are destroyed by freezing or boiling.

Toxicity Signs/Symptoms:

Occurs 2-6 hours after ingestion; nausea, vomiting, diarrhea, oral irritation; renal damage may occur.

Treatment:

First Aid – First, emesis then milk or water to dilute and decontaminate; charcoal; cold water or ice for mouth.

Medical – Gastric lavage; cathartic; IV calcium gluconate for tetany or hypocalacemia.

Other – Check urine for oxalate crystals; monitor serum calcium, BUN, and creatinine; maintain adequate urine flow with hydration.

References:

5, 6, 14, 104, 107

Ruta graveolens L.   Rutaceae

Common Names:

Rue, herb of grace, German rue

Parts Containing Toxins:

Leaves and unripened fruit, especially when fresh.

Toxic Constituents – Oil with 2-nonanone, limonene (volatile oils); bergapten, xanthotoxin, psoralen (furanocoumarins).

Doses:

Therapeutic – Powder 65-648 mg; tincture 1-10 drops (0.06-0.62 ml); oil 1-6 drops (0.06-0.37 ml).

Lethal – Oil LD_{50} 2.5-5.0 gm/kg orally.

Note:

Contraindications – In pregnancy due to its emmenagogue and human abortifacient effects from its uterine stimulant alkaloid skimmianine. Avoid exposure to ultraviolet light or sun for 12 hours after topical application.

Mechanism of Toxicity – The volatile oil in rue is a gastrointestinal irritant and destructive to the nervous system. The furanocoumarins in the oil are phototoxic, especially when used externally.

Toxicity Signs/Symptoms:

Internal – Narcosis, melacholic moods, sleep disorders, tiredness; violent gastric pains, nausea, vomiting, dizziness, spasms; irritation to mucosa, renal irritation and damage, liver degeneration; prostration, confusion, delirium, fainting, tremor, spasms, convulsions, death.

External – Phototoxic reactions are possible. Contact dermitits, burning, redness, vesiculation.

Treatment:

First Aid – Emesis; activated charcoal; for dermatitis, wash the exposed area well twice with soap and water.

Medical – Gastric lavage if no emesis; cathartic; monitor and replace fluid and electrolytes.

References:

3, 5, 9, 11, 14, 25, 100, 104, 105, 106, 107

S

Sambucus canadensis L.,
Sambucus nigra L.   **Caprifoliaceae**

Common Names:

Elder, elderberry, ellanwood, ellhorn

Parts Containing Toxins:

Leaves, shoots, bark and roots, seeds, raw unripe berries.

Toxic Constituents – Sambunigrin (cyanogenic glycoside).

Doses:

Therapeutic – Tincture 20-40 drops (1.23-2.47 ml).

Note:

Mechanism of Toxicity – The glycoside in large amounts can produce cyanide poisoning, with resultant cellular hypoxia.

Other – Cooking destroys the toxins.

Flowers, the medicinal part most commonly used, are nontoxic.

Toxicity Signs/Symptoms:

Dizziness, headache, nausea, vomiting, gastrointestinal distress, diarrhea, tachycardia, convulsions.

Treatment:

Medical – Charcoal, after gastric lavage, preceded by endotracheal intubation; cathartic; amyl nitrite under nose or mouth 30 seconds each minute; IV sodium nitrite, followed with sodium thiosulfate; IV diazepam for seizures; emergency exchange transfusion for methemoglobinemia.

References:

1, 5, 7, 8, 12, 14, 104, 106

Sanguinaria canadensis L.   Papaveraceae

Common Names:

Bloodroot, red puccon, red root, Indian paint, tetterwort paucon, coon root, snakebite, sweet slumber

Parts Containing Toxins:

Rhizomes, all parts.

Toxic Constituents – 1% Sanguinarine, chelerythrine (isoquinoline alkaloids), berberine, coptisine (protoberberine alkaloids) and others.

Doses:

Therapeutic – Root powder 64.8-324 mg;

tincture 5-20 drops (0.31-1.23 ml);

fluid extract 1-10 drops (0.06-0.62 ml).

Toxic – Root powder 175 mg.

Lethal – Alkaloids from methanolic and hydromethanolic

extracts LD_{50} 1440 and 1250 mg/kg orally in rats, respectively; sanguinarine LD_{50} 1658 mg/kg orally in rats.

Note:

Contraindications – In pregnancy since it is an emmenagogue and may be abortifacient. It contains the animal uterine stimulant alkaloids berberine, protopine, and chelerythrine.

Mechanism of Toxicity – This plant acts as a gastric irritant and emetic, causing severe cramping followed by local paralysis.

Toxicity Signs/Symptoms:

Internal – Burning gastralgia, nausea, diaphoresis, increased expectoration, vomiting, diarrhea, intestinal colic; diminished or disordered vision, dizziness, headaches and vertigo, muscular relaxation, marked thirst, dilated pupils and slow irregular cardiac action; cold extremities; burning sensation, fainting; also, prostration, shock, coma, convulsions, death by cardiac and respiratory failure.

Also, allergic angioedema has been reported.

External – Contact dermatitis when handled fresh.

Treatment:

First Aid – Emesis; charcoal; strong tea. For dermatitis, wash twice with soap and water.

Medical – Gastric lavage if no emesis; opiates to allay GI irritation and pain; cathartic; maintain fluid and electrolyte balance.

Other – Demulcents.

References:

1, 3, 7, 9, 10, 12, 14, 25, 68, 100, 103, 104, 107, 180, 181

Selenicereus grandiflorus (L.) Britton & Rose.
(= *Cactus grandiflorus* L.)   Cactaceae

Common Names:

Night-blooming cereus, large-flowered cactus, sweet-scented cactus, vanilla cactus

Parts Containing Toxins:

Flowers and fresh green stems.

Toxic Constituents – Hordenine (alkaloid).

Doses:

Therapeutic – Tincture 5-30 drops (0.31-1.85 ml); fluid extract 1-20 drops (0.06-1.23 ml).

Note:

Kinetics – Hordenine is absorbed intact and de-aminated in the liver by monoamine oxidase B.

Mechanism of Toxicity – Hordenine is an adrenergic alkaloid that potentiates contractions on circular myocardial fibers and is a sympathetic stimulant to the cardiac plexus. It acts by inhibiting norepinephrine uptake.

Other – The species *Selenicereus pteranthus* also contains hordenine and has at times been used as a substitute.

Toxicity Signs/Symptoms:

Tachycardia, arrhythmia, cardiospasm, mental confusion, violent throbbing headaches, hyperesthesia, vertigo, amblyopia and gastrointestinal upset; quickened pulse, constricted sensation in chest, sensitive to noise; sadness or paranoia, followed by melancholy; carditis, pericarditis.

Treatment:

(See Treatment section under Explanation of Format.)

References:

3, 9, 10, 127, 128

Senecio aureus L.,
Senecio spp.   **Asteraceae**

Common Names:

Life root, golden senecio, cocash weed, squaw weed; ragwort

Parts Containing Toxins:

Whole herb.

Toxic Constituents –Senecionine, seneciphylline, jacobine and more than 40 others (pyrrolizidine alkaloids) in most species and florosensine, otosenine, and floridanine (pyrrolizidine alkaloids) in *S. aureus.*

Doses:

Therapeutic – Powdered herb 3.2-3.89 gm.

Note:

Contraindications – In pregnancy due to the teratogenic and uterine stimulant effects of the genus and the emmenagogue and abortifacient effects of *S. aureus. Senecio* spp. should not be used internally due to their potential hepatotoxicity.

Mechanism of Toxicity – Pyrrolizidines are the only known hepatotoxic alkaloids. In addition to necrodegenerative hepatitis, they produce hypertensive pulmonary vascular disease. It is thought to have a hindering effect at neuromuscular junctions.

Other – It is most toxic in its young stages; North American species are less toxic than African.

Children appear to be more sensitive to hepatotoxic effects.

Studies of *Senecio jacobaea* (tansy ragwort) show hepatotoxicity is potentiated by copper. *S. jacobaea* is teratogenic, also.

Toxicity Signs/Symptoms:

Acute – Hepatic enlargement and necrosis and collagenous occlusion of small branches of venous tree (venoocclusive disease), progressing to a nonportal cirrhosis; ascites, abdominal pain, nausea and vomiting, headache.

Chronic – Emaciation, progressive lesions of liver and lungs; may lead to hepatocarcinoma diagnosed by biopsy; also, ascites, enlarged liver, apathy.

Treatment:

First Aid – [Acute] Emesis; activated charcoal; for dermatitis, wash twice.

Medical – [Acute] Gastric lavage if no emesis; cathartic; maintain fluid and electrolyte balance.

Other – [Acute/Chronic] Remove from source; support liver function.

References:

2, 6, 8, 11, 12, 14, 19, 20, 25, 28, 34, 47, 48, 104, 106, 107, 113, 114

Solanum dulcumara L.;
Solanum nigrum L.   Solanaceae

Common Names:

Bittersweet, woody nightshade, scarlet berry, violet bloom, felonwort, fever twig; black nightshade, garden nightshade, poisonberry

Parts Containing Toxins:

Leaves and fruit (especially unripened fruit).

Toxic Constituents – Solanine, solasonine, demissine and others (glycosidal alkaloids). Dulcamarinic acid and dulcamarstinic acid (steroidal saponins) in *S. dulcumara*.

Doses:

Therapeutic – *S. dulcumara* tincture 10-15 drops (0.62-0.93 ml).

Toxic – 10 Berries.

Lethal – 200 Beries.

Note:

Kinetics – Solanine is hydrolized in the gut to free alkamines such as the less toxic solanidine. Solanine is poorly absorbed from the GI tract and is rapidly excreted in the urine and feces. Tissue peak levels occur after 12 hours.

Mechanism of Toxicity – The alkaloids can affect the CNS with anticholinergic effects. However, solanine inhibits cholinesterase. The saponins are strong irritants to the mucosa.

Other – The symptoms appear a few hours after ingestion, or may take 12-24 hours to appear.

The 2-3 year old twigs without leaves and sometimes the bark of the root of *S. dulcumara* are used medicinally and the toxins in these parts are relatively weak. However, excessive use of the stems (over 25 gm) has led to poisoning. The leaves and whole plant of *S. nigrum* are normally used and can cause serious effects, though usually not fatal.

Toxicity Signs/Symptoms:

Salivation, lowered temperature, burning in throat, nausea, dizziness, dilated pupils; slow or rapid heart rate, rapid breathing, abdominal pain, vomiting, diarrhea, mental and respiratory depression; dulling of senses; hypothermia or fever, headache, delirium, skin hot and dry, shock, rigid extremities, tremors, convulsive movements, pain in joints, erythematous eruptions, stupefaction, depressed respiration and circulation; also, stomach pain, itching in mouth; collapse, coma and death from paralysis.

Treatment:

First Aid – Establish respiration; emesis; activated charcoal.

Medical – If anticholinergic crisis symptoms, physystigmine 0.2-2.0 mg (0.02 mg/kg) slow intravenous push repeat as necessary; gastric lavage if no emesis; cathartic; maintain fluids with appropriate IV solution to help establish electrolyte balance; IV diazepam for seizures; alkalinize blood and give propranolol for arrhythmias.

References:

1, 3, 5, 6, 7, 8, 9, 10, 14, 101, 103, 104, 106, 107, 182

Spigelia marilandica L.   Loganiaceae

Common Names:

Pinkroot, Maryland pink, Carolina pink, worm grass, starbloom

Parts Containing Toxins:

Root and rhizome.

Toxic Constituents – Spigeline (alkaloid).

Doses:

Therapeutic – Powder 2-5 grams; tincture 15-39 drops (0.93-2.41 ml); fluid extract 5-60 drops (0.31-3.7 ml).

Note:

Other – Use of the root to paralyze worms is followed by a strong laxative to expel them.

Toxicity Signs/Symptoms:

Increased cardiac action; cerebral disturbance, dizziness, dimness of vision, dilated pupils, facial and palpebral spasms, purgation, general convulsions and stupor; possibly

death through asphyxiation.

Prolonged use has depressive effects upon the heart.

Treatment:

(See Treatment section in Explanation of Format.)

References:

3, 6, 9, 100, 104, 107

Stillingia sylvatica Garden ex L.   Euphorbiaceae

Common Names:

Queen's root, queen's-delight, cockup hat, marcory, silver leaf

Parts Containing Toxins:

Dried root (less than 1 year old).

Toxic Constituents – Sylvacrol (alcohol), prostatin, gnidilatidin, and others (diterpene esters).

Doses:

Therapeutic – Powder 0.32-3.89 grams; tincture 1-60 drops (0.06-3.7 ml); fluid extract 1-30 drops (0.06-1.85 ml).

Note:

Mechanism of Toxicity – The fresh plant and root are skin and strong mucous membrane irritants.

Other – Handling the fresh root can lead to inflammation and swelling.

Toxicity Signs/Symptoms:

Gastroenteritis with severe burning; heavy, bile-filled, loose diarrhea; vomiting, tachycardia and muscular weakness, prostration.

Treatment:

Use demulcents to alleviate gastrointestinal discomfort.

References:

3, 9, 100, 104, 107, 110

Strophanthus hispidus DC., *Strophanthus kombe* Oliver   **Apocynaceae**

Common Names:

Strophanthus

Parts Containing Toxins:

Dried ripe seed.

Toxic Constituents – 4.0-4.5% K-strophanthin (steroid glycoside).

Doses:

Therapeutic – Tincture 5-15 drops (0.31-0.93 ml).

Note:

Precautions – Simultaneous use of quinidine, calcium salts, and potassium-lowing drugs including thiazide diuretics, laxatives, licorice, and glucocorticoids increase the potential for adverse effects.

Contraindications – In pregancy since it is a potential abortifacient due to its animal uterine stimulant activity. Also avoid in myocardial degeneration, extensive valvular lesions, peripheral vascular disease of arteriosclerosis, atheromas and aneurisms.

Mechanism of Toxicity – Strophanthin is a myogenic cardiac stimulant whose action is rapid (onset 5-10 minutes; peak effect 30-120 minutes).

Toxicity Signs/Symptoms:

GI irritation with vomiting and diarrhea; muscles enfeebled, then rigid fibrillary twitchings; headache, stupor, disturbance of color vision, cardiac arrhythmias; finally, pallid, noncontractile and hard rigor mortis of heart and body; cardiospasm; frequent brief systole followed by enormous increase in blood pressure; cessation of heart in systole; respiration ceases last; death.

Treatment:

First Aid – CPR; emetics quickly; activated charcoal.

Medical – Atropine 0.6 mg IV for bradycardia; epsom salt purge; monitor serum potassium, and for hyperkalemia give Kayeralate (R) or glucose/ insulin; phenytoin or transvenous electrical pacemaker for complete heart block.

References:

3, 6, 7, 9, 10, 14, 25, 103, 107

Strychnos ignatia Lind.   **Loganiaceae**

Common Names:

St. Ignatius bean, faba ignatii

Parts Containing Toxins:

Seed, whole herb.

Toxic Constituents – 2-3% Strychnine, 1-1.5% brucine and others (indole alkaloids); igasuric acid; loganin (glycosides).

Doses:

Therapeutic – Powder 32.4-64.8 mg; tincture 0.5-5 drops (0.03-0.31 ml).

Toxic – 1 Seed; strychnine 5 mg.

Lethal – Powder 1-2 gm; strychnine 30-90 mg, 15 mg in small child.

Note:

Precautions – Prolonged use should be avoided.

Kinetics – Absorbed rapidly by GI tract; metabolized in 24 hours by the liver; excreted in the urine. Strychnine is cumulative, especially if there is liver damage.

Mechanism of Toxicity – CNS stimulation by selective blocks on motor inhibitors at the postsynaptic membrane in the ventral horns of the spinal column (the primary effect).

Other – See *Strychnos nux-vomica* for additional toxicity information.

Toxicity Signs/Symptoms:

Prodrome – Muscle cramps, stiffness, agitation.

Acute – Convulsions begin in 15-60 minutes; lactic acidemia, spasms, opisthotonos, respiratory compromise with death due to hypoxia.

Chronic – Subconvulsive doses over several weeks can lead to death under similar circumstances. Liver damage is caused by drug accumulation.

Lab – Elevated SGOT, LDH, and CPK; leucocytosis.

Treatment:

First Aid – Empty stomach quickly by emesis. Activated charcoal or tannins.

Medical – Gastric lavage (contraindicated once seizures have begun) with dilute potassium permanganate or iodide, then promptly removed from the stomach. Saline cathartic. Monitor arterial blood gases; high calorie glucose infusions; IV sodium bicarbonate for acidemia. IV diazepam or barbital for seizures; curare with mechanical ventilation if refractory convulsions.

Other – Keep patient quiet, recumbent, protected from draughts and in a dark room. Belladonna, aconite, or tobacco may be tried. Analeptics or phenothiazines should not be given.

References:

3, 7, 9, 14, 103, 107

Strychnos nux-vomica L.   **Loganiaceae**

Common Names:

Quaker' s buttons, nux vomica, poison nut

Parts Containing Toxins:

Dried ripened seeds, whole herb.

Toxic Constituents – 1-2% Strychnine and brucine, along with vomicine and others (indole alkaloids); loganin (glycoside); caffeotannic acid.

Doses:

Therapeutic – Powder 3.24-129.6 mg; tincture 1-15 drops (0.06-0.93 ml).

Toxic – Strychnine 5 mg.

Lethal – Powder 1.94 grams; 1 seed; strychnine 30-90 mg or 15 mg in small child.

Note:

Contraindications – In pregnancy due to its emmenagogue and probable abortifacient effects.

Kinetics – Absorbed rapidly by GI tract; metabolized in 24 hours by the liver; excreted in the urine. Strychnine is cumulative, especially if there is liver damage.

Mechanism of Toxicity – Strychnine causes CNS stimulation by selective blocks on motor inhibitors at the postsynaptic membrane in the ventral horns of the spinal column as its primary effect. This increases reflex excitability.

Other – The symptoms occur 10-60 minutes after ingestion.

If death does not occur after 6 hours, recovery is likely.

Toxicity Signs/Symptoms:

Uneasiness and restlessness, dysphagia, anoxia, cyanosis, paraesthesia, tachycardia, hyperhydrosis. Sense of impending suffocation, tremors of whole body; sudden convulsions of great violence, opisthotonos, risus sardonicus. Convulsions are followed by rest period with pain, weariness and rending of limbs, acute sensibility and dreadful alarm; the slightest stimulus will renew convulsions. Death occurs in 2 hours after 2-5 convulsions as a result of exhaustion or paralytic asphyxia; rigor mortis persists for months.

Lab – Elevated SGOT, LDH, and CPK; leucocytosis.

Treatment:

First Aid – CPR with firm contact (sensitive to light touch); activated charcoal. Keep patient absolutely quiet.

Medical – Emesis or gastric lavage only before symptoms begin; after symptoms appear emesis or gastric lavage may induce convulsions; lavage with potassium permanganate or iodine and tannins; concentration of neutralizers should be tannic acid 2%, iodine tincture in water (1:250), and potassium permanganate (1:5000). Saline cathartic; amyl nitrate; monitor arterial blood gases; high calorie glucose infusions; treat acidemia with IV sodium bicarbonate; for seizures use IV diazepam or barbital; curare with mechanical ventilation and oxygen if refractory convulsions.

Other – Keep them recumbent, in a quiet, darkened room and protected from draughts.

References:

3, 6, 7, 9, 13, 14, 25, 103, 106, 107

Symphytum officinale L.;
Symphytum x uplandicum Nyman.   **Boraginaceae**

Common Names:

Comfrey, knitbone, knitback, blackwort, bruisewort, slippery root, wallwort; Russian comfrey

Parts Containing Toxins:

Roots and leaves.

Toxic Constituents – Symphytine, echimidine, 7-acetyl-lycopsamine, and others (pyrrolizidine alkaloids and N-oxides).

Doses:

Therapeutic – External use only, not to exceed 100 mcg toxic pyrrolizidine alkaoids daily.

Toxic – Leaf 8% of diet; root 1% of diet for 2/3-1 2/3 years (in rats). Alkaloids 40 ug/kg/day for 2 years (human equivalent of 2 leaves/day for 2 years).

Note:

Precautions – Internal use should be avoided due to potential for hepatotoxic and carcinogenic effects of alkaloids. Also, avoid use on skin that is not intact due to burns, abrasions or lacerations. (Percutaneous absorption leaves the N-oxides intact. Minimal alkaloidal absorption occurs through intact skin.)

Contraindications – In pregnancy and lactation due to possible liver damage to the infant.

Mechanism of Toxicity – The pyrrolizidine alkaloid-N-oxides with 1,2-unsaturated necine structure are reduced by gut bacteria to the free alkaloids. The alkaloids are metabolised by mixed-function oxidases in the liver to reactive pyrrolic dehydro-alkaloids.

Other – The effects are cumulative and overt damage may be long delayed.

Do not used externally for more than 4-6 weeks per year.

Other medicinal plants in the Boraginaceae family containing toxic pyrrolizidines that should be avoided, especially during pregnancy, include *Alkanna tinctoria* (alkanet), *Heliotropium europaeum* (heliotrope), and *Borago officinalis* (borage).

Toxicity Signs/Symptoms:

Chronic – Several cases of veno-occlusive disease of the liver leading to fatigue, diarrhea,weight loss, fever, abdominal pain, hepatomegaly, ascites, and portal hypertension due to obliteration of small hepatic veins.

Development of cancers in various organs, especially hepatocellular adenomas, and pulmonary endothelial hyperplasia (in rats).

Lab – Hyperbilirubinemia, elevated alkaline phosphate, and SGOT.

X-rays – Reticulonodular shadowing in mid-zone and base of lung.

Treatment:

Cease internal comfrey use and assess and treat for liver damage.

References:

5, 14, 24, 26, 27, 29, 31, 33, 48, 100, 106, 107, 183, 184, 185

T

Tanacetum vulgare L.   Asteraceae

Common Names:

Tansy, bitter buttons, hindheal, parsley fern

Parts Containing Toxins:

Leaves and tops.

Toxic Constituents – Oil with thujone, beta-isothujone, borneol, camphor (volatile ketones) and tanacetin (sesquiterpene lactone).

Doses:

Therapeutic – Oil 1-10 drops (0.05-0.50 ml); powder 0.32-3.89 grams; tincture 1-30 drops (0.06-1.85 ml).

Toxic – Oil > 15 drops (0.75 ml) is dangerous; thujone 30 mg/kg body weight.

Lethal – Oil 4 ml, oral LD_{50} 0.30 gm/kg in dogs and 1.15 gm/kg in rats; thujone LD_{50} 0.21 orally in animals.

Note:

Contraindications – In pregnancy due to its emmenagogue, abortifacient and animal uterine stimulant effects. The oil should not be used internally or externally in therapy.

Toxicity Signs/Symptoms:

Gastroenteritis, nausea, vomiting, diarrhea, cramps, abdominal pain, flushing, mydriasis; uterine bleeding, increased pulse rate, weak pulse, irregular heartbeat, rapid breathing; severe reddening of face, dilated and rigid pupils, convulsions, paralysis, tonic-clonic spasms, frothing from mouth, kidney damage, hepatitis; also coma, death by respiratory paralysis after 1-3.5 hours.

External – Dermatitis in those who are sensitive to Asteracea plants.

Treatment:

First Aid – Activated charcoal; cathartic; avoid oils and alcohol; for dermatitis, wash twice.

Medical – Gastric lavage; monitor cardiac function closely; prevent aspiration pneumonitis; for seizures give IV diazepam. Do lipid hemodialysis or resin hemoperfusion if severe neurologic or respiratory symptoms fail to respond to standard supportive care.

References:

2, 3, 5, 6, 8, 9, 11, 12, 14, 25, 100, 104, 105, 107

Taxus spp.   Taxaceae

Common Names:

Yew, chinwood

Parts Containing Toxins:

Leaves, seeds, bark.

Toxic Constituents – Taxines A and B (pseudoalkaloids), biflavonoids and cyanogenic glycosides.

Doses:

Therapeutic – Mother tincture 5 drops (0.3 ml).

Lethal – Fresh needles 50-100 gm.

Note:

Contraindications – In pregnancy due to use as an emmenagogue and abortifacient.

Kinetics – Taxine is rapidly absorbed from the intestines. Symptoms appear a few hours after ingestion.

Mechanism of Toxicity – Taxines are cardiac depressants. Taxine B inhibits calcium and sodium transport in myocardial cells.

Other – The part of the plant usually consumed by children in reported "poisonings" are the fruits which are not poisonous.

The cancer chemotherapeutic compounds taxol (paclitaxel) from the bark of *Taxus brevifolia* and the semisynthetic docetaxel from *Taxus baccata* needles are not present in nature in effective therapeutic quantities. For example, taxol is in *Taxus* x *media* cultivar "Hicksi" fresh needles at 0.0086-0.0094 gm% and in microwave dried and vacuum dried needles at 0.0052 and 0.0029 gm%, respectively, and in "Dark Green Spreader" cultivar room temperature dried and barn-dried needles at 0.0067-0.0092 and 0.0047-0.0138 gm%, respectively.

Toxicity Signs/Symptoms:

Nausea, vomiting, abdominal pain, dizziness, tachycardia; bradycardia, hypotension, nervousness, muscular weakness, trembling, dyspnea, dilated pupils, reddened lips, incoordination, confusion, convulsions, respiratory depression, coma; death is sudden due to asphyxiation or cardiac failure from rhythm distubances. Bradycardia indicates a poor prognosis.

Treatment:

First Aid – Emesis if immediately after accidental consumption; activated charcoal.

Medical – Gastric lavage with potassium permanganate if no emesis; saline cathartic; IV diazepam or barbital for seizures; plasma volume expanders for shock; lidocaine for cardiac rhythm disorders. Transvenous cardiac pacing for bradycardia; mechanical ventilation with oxygen if necessary. Monitor kidney function, blood coagulation and liver values.

References:

6, 7, 103, 104, 107, 186, 187, 188, 189, 190, 191

Teucrium chamaedrys L.   Lamiaceae

Common Names:

Germander, common germander, wall germander

Parts Containing Toxins:

Flowering plant.

Toxic Constituents – Teucrins, teuflin, teucvin and others (neo-clerodane diterpenoids).

Doses:

Toxic – Powder 0.26-1.6 gm per day for 2-18 weeks.

Note:

Contraindications – Due to serious toxic risk compared to negligible benefits, germander should not be used therapeutically.

Mechanism of Toxicity – Acute hepatitis develops with continued exposure to diterpenoid metabolites whose metabolites deplete cellular thiols, especially glutathione.

amino acids and by inducing activity of 3A family of cytochrome P-450 with dexamethasone.

The American species *Teucrium canadensis* known as "pink" skullcap contains the neo-clerodane diterpenoids isoteuflin, teuflin, teucvin and others and is frequently sold simply as skullcap in Great Britain. This spurious substitution is probably responsible for European hepatotoxic reports associated with the American "blue" skullcap (*Scutellaria lateriflora*).

Toxicity Signs/Symptoms:

Acute – Nausea, stomach pain, dyspepsia.

Chronic – Nausea or vomiting, jaundice, weakness, abdominal pain, dark urine, fever, itching, hepatomegaly, death with continual consumption.

Lab – Elevated AST (SGOT), ALT (SGPT), and alkaline phosphatase; decreased prothrombin, hypereosinophilia. Hepatic necrosis with inflammatory infiltration and fibrous portal tracts have been found on biopsy.

Treatment:

Medical – Induce glutathione conjugate formation and prevent glutathione depletion with cystine. Stop germander intake; jaundice disappears within 8 weeks.

References:

100, 101, 102, 107, 192, 193, 194, 195, 196, 197, 198

Thuja occidentalis L.   Cupressaceae

Common Names:

Arbor vitae, tree of life, northern white cedar, eastern white cedar, swamp cedar, yellow cedar, hackmatack

Parts Containing Toxins:

Leaves and twigs.

Toxic Constituents – 1.4-4% Oil with 31-65% alpha-thujone and 7-15% beta-thujone (volatile ketones).

Doses:

Therapeutic – Tincture 1-30 drops (0.06-1.85 ml).

Toxic – Oil 30 mg/kg body weight; 1 ml twice daily for 5 days.

Lethal – Oil LD_{50} 0.83 gm/kg orally in animals; thujone LD_{50} 0.21 gm/kg orally in animals.

Note:

Contraindications – In pregnancy since it has been used as an emmenagogue and a human abortifacient. The oil should not be used internally.

Mechanism of Toxicity – Thujone is neurotoxic to the CNS and a cardiac stimulant.

Other – Alpha-thujone is more toxic than beta-thujone. Though the oil of western red cedar, *Thuja plicata,* contains less alpha- than beta-thujone (5-10% and 70-80%, respectively), it also has a potentially severe neurotoxicity and should not be used therapeutically.

Toxicity Signs/Symptoms:

Acute – Nausea, vomiting, gastroenteritis, mucosal hemorrhages, flatulence; convulsions associated with lesions of the cerebral cortex; decreased blood pressure, painful diarrhea; coma and death.

Chronic – Renal damage and personality change.

Treatment:

First Aid – Establish respiration; emesis; activated charcoal.

Medical – Gastric lavage with potassium permanganate if no emesis; saline cathartic; monitor cardiac function closely; avoid aspiration pneumonitis; for seizures use IV diazepam; atropine for colic; replace electrolytes; sodium bicarbonate for acidosis; monitor kidney function; mechanical ventilation with oxygen if necessary.

Other – Keep rested, quiet and warm.

References:

2, 3, 5, 9, 14, 25, 100, 104, 105, 107

Toxicodendron radicans (L.) Kuntze (= *Rhus toxicodendron* L.) Anacardiaceae

Common Names:

Poison ivy, poison vine

Parts Containing Toxins:

Leaves and branches, whole plant.

Toxic Constituents – Urushiol (oleoresin containing 3-n-pentadecylcatechol) .

Doses:

Therapeutic – Powder 0.03-0.05 gm; tincture 1-5 drops (0.06-0.31 ml).

Note:

Contraindications – In pregnancy due to its uterine stimulant activity.

Mechanism of Toxicity – Sensitivity to urushiol induces production of immunoregulatory proteins and T lymphocyte activation on exposure.

Other – Contact dermatitis from plants can occur with live or dead material. Inhaling smoke from burning poison ivy plants has been associated with respiratory distress syndrome.

Toxicity Signs/Symptoms:

External – Itching, burning, redness and vesiculation; coated tongue, headache and delirium; secondary infection from scratching or moist applications.

Internal – Mucosal inflammation, colic, diarrhea, drowsiness, stupor, vomiting, vertigo, impairment of special senses, mydriasis, chilliness, nausea, thirst, burning pain, feeling of constriction in the temporal region; pulse slow, weakness trembling, stupor, kidney damage with hematuria, swelling, fever; unconsciousness, death.

Treatment:

First Aid – (For internal exposure) Emesis, activated charcoal.

(For contact dermatitis) Wash with soapy water and then clean with ethanol. Cover inflammationw with sodium bicarbonate mixed with water to make a paste.

Medical – (For internal exposure) Gastric lavage with potassium permanganate if no emesis; saline cathartic; IV diazepam for spasms; plasma volume expanders for shock, keep warm and quiet; sodium bicarbonate for acidosis; monitor kidney function; mechanical ventilation with oxygen if necessary.

(For contact dermatitis) Oral corticosteroids. Immunity may be strengthened with subcutaneous injection or oral administration of an extract of the plant itself.

Other – (For contact dermatitis) Thin cloths soaked in cool water are applied locally with or without extracts of *Impatiens pallida* and *I. fulva*, *Oenothera biennis*, *Quercus alba*, *Lobelia inflata*, *Baptisia tinctoria*, *Hydrastis canadensis*, *Hamamelis virginica*, or fresh bark of *Alnus serrulata* or a combination thereof.

References:

6, 7, 8, 9, 10, 12, 14, 25, 105, 107, 199

Tussilago farfara L.   Asteraceae

Common Names:

Coltsfoot, coughwort, foal's foot, horsehoof, hallfoot, foalswort, fieldhove

Parts Containing Toxins:

Flower buds, leaves, root.

Toxic constituents – Senkirkine, tussilagine, and possibly

others (pyrrolizidine alkaloids) total 0.004-0.03% in flowers and
0.005% in leaves.

Doses:

Therapeutic – Leaves at maximum 10 mcg pyrrolizidine
alkaloids per day, or 1 mcg per day for maximum of 4-6 weeks
per year.

Toxic – Flower buds as 8% or more of diet of rats as carcinogen.

Note:

Contraindications –In pregnancy due to its potential
abortifacient effect (including root) and potential hepatotoxic
effect on fetus. Nursing mothers should also avoid its use.

Mechanism of Action – The pyrrolizidine alkaloids are
hepatotoxic, causing veno-occlusive disease with centrilobular
fibrosis and connective tissue occlusion of small and medium size
hapatic veins. The alkaloids are also genotoxic and carcinogenic
with prolonged use.

Other – Certain closely-related Asteraceae plants including
Petasites spp. have similar pyrrolizidine alkaloid constituents such
as the senecionine. Their effects and contraindications should be
considered the same. The similar appearing leaves of the plant
Adenostyles alliariae containing the pyrrolizidine alkaloid
senecipylline and its N-oxide were mistakenly picked and used as
coltsfoolt, resulting in a case of veno-occlusive disease in an
infant. Absolute identification of *Tussilago farfara* in toxicity
cases involving humans has not been made. The leaves are the
part normally used in medicine in the West. The higher
concentration of alkaloids in the flowers should be avoided.

Toxicity Signs/Symptoms:

Chronic – Hepatomegaly and ascites. In rats
hemangioendothelial sarcoma in the liver.

Treatment:

Stop use of plant. Assess and treat hepatotoxic effects.

References:

25, 100, 101, 106, 107, 114, 200, 201, 202

U

Urginea maritima (L.) Baker,
Urginea indica Kunth   Liliaceae

Common Names:

White squill, sea onion, squill, scilla, drimia

Parts Containing Toxins:

Dried inner fleshy scales.

Toxic Constituents – Scillarin A and B, proscillaridin A (bufadienolides) and about two dozen other glycosides.

Doses:

Therapeutic – Powder 64.8-194.4 mg; tincture 5-30 drops (0.31-1.85 ml).

Note:

Contraindications – In potassium deficiency or when digitalis glycosides are being used. Also avoid in second or third degree atrioventricular blocks, hypercalcemia, hypertrophic cardiomyopathy, carotid sinus syndrome, ventricular tachycardia, thoracic aortic aneurysm and Wolff-Parkinson-White syndrome.

Kinetics – Between 20-30% of the cardioactive glycosides are absorbed. Their half-lives are from 23-49 hours, and the duration of activity is from 2-3 days. About 85% are protein bound, and they are mainly excreted through the liver.

Mechanism of Toxicity – Squill has a cardiac and GI influence similar to digitalis. It is positively inotropic and negatively chronotropic.

Other – Do not confuse with the red variety of *Urginea maritima* which is used as a rat poison.

Increases toxicity when used with quinidine, calcium, diuretics, laxatives and glucocorticoids.

Increased risk of cardiac arrhythmias when combined with

symphathomimetics, methylxanthine alkaloids, phosphodiesterase inhibitors or quinidine.

Toxicity Signs/Symptoms:

Gastrointestinal irritation, nausea, vomiting, abdominal cramps and diarrhea, loss of appetite; headache, acute congestive nephritis with albuminuria, hematuria, diminished renal output or anuria; irregular pulse, ventricular tachycardia, atrial tachycardia with AV-block; vision disorders, dullness and stupor, confusion, hallucinations, psychosis; intermittent paralysis and convulsions, death in 10-24 hours by asphyxiation, gastroenteritis, nephritis, or cardiac block.

Treatment:

First Aid – Emesis; activated charcoal.

Medical – Gastric lavage if no emesis; cathartic; atropine 0.6 mg IV; monitor serum potassium; for hyperkalemia giveKayeralate (R) or glucose/insulin; for heart block give phenytoin or use transvenous electrical pacemaker; lidocaine for ventricular extrsystole; atropine for bradycaridia; hemoperfusion to eliminate glycosides or cholestyramine to interupt enterhepatic circulation.

References:

3, 6, 7, 9, 14, 93, 106, 107

V

Valeriana officinalis L.   Valerianaceae

Common Names:

Valerian, all-heal, heliotrope, setwall, vandal root

Parts Containing Toxins:

Root and rhizome.

Toxic Constituents – 0.2-1.0% Volatile oil with valeranone; 0.1-0.9% valerenic acids (volatile sesquiterpenes), isovaltrate, didrovaltrate, and others (valepotriates 0.2-2.0%).

Doses:

Therapeutic – Tincture 0.5-1.0 tsp (1.85-3.7 ml); fluid extract 10-20 drops (0.62-1.23 ml); oil 1-5 drops (0.06-0.31 ml).

Toxic – Powder 40 capsules (470 mg each); valerenic acid 150-200 mg/kg IP in mice.

Lethal - Valerenic acid 400 mg/kg IP in mice; valepotriates LD_{50} 64-150 mg/kg IP in mice. (Valepotriates <u>not</u> toxic at 4.6 gm/kg orally in mice).

Note:

Precaution – Use may affect driving ability.

Toxicity Signs/Symptoms:

Acute – Headache, giddiness, perverted vision, restlessness, agitation, nausea; decreased sensibility, motility and reflex excitability; central paralysis; fatigue, abdominal cramps and pain, chest tightness, tremors, light headedness.

Chronic – Headache, restlessness, sleeplessness, dilated pupils, cardiac dysfunction.

Treatment:

First Aid – Activated charcoal.

References:

10, 46, 101, 102, 106, 107

Veratrum album L.;
Veratrum viride Aiton.   **Liliaceae**

Common Names:

White hellebore, European hellebore; green hellebore, American hellebore, swamp hellebore, Indian poke, itch weed, bugbane, devil's bite, earth gall

Parts Containing Toxins:

Roots and rhizome, all parts.

Toxic Constituents – Protoveratrine A & B (steroid alkaloids); veratrine, veratridine, veratramine, veratrasine, veratrin (glycoalkaloids).

Doses:

Therapeutic – Root powder 65-130 mg; tincture 2-10 drops (0.12-0.62ml); fluid extract 1-3 drops (0.06-0.18 ml).

Toxic – Fresh parts 1 gram.

Lethal – Powder 1-2 gm; alkaloids 10-20 mg.

Note:

Contraindications – In pregnancy due to teratogenic effects of the alkaloids. The nonmedicinal species *Veratrum californicum* and *Veratrum eschscholtizii* have been found to be teratogenic due to their cyclopamine, jervine, and cycloposine content.

Kinetics – The alkaloids act within 2 hours and the effects persist 4-6 hours; they're degraded in the liver and excreted in the feces.

Mechanism of Toxicity – The alkaloids act by afferent sympathetic stimulation, slowing the heart and lowering blood pressure by vagus reflex in the heart and lungs, and also dilate the arterioles. Afferent cardiac and coronary receptor stimulation transmitted by the vagus nerve reflexly lowers blood pressure and heart rate, known as the Bezold-Jarisch reflex. The alkaloids increase sodium conductivity with secondary loss of potassium leading to a decreased threshold for stimulation for nerves and muscles. Large doses raise the blood pressure by direct effect on vasomotor center. The root is also a strong irritant to the skin and mucosa.

Other – Poisoning is seldom fatal due to rapid vomiting and poor intestinal absorption.

Large amounts may cause death, but only a small amount is necessary to produce symptoms.

Most potent in the spring. Sometimes mistakenly gathered and cooked as a vegetable.

Toxicity Signs/Symptoms:

    Acute – Burning in mouth, fauces, pharynx and stomach; sneezing, lacrimation, salivation, nausea, severe vomiting, diarrhea, muscular weakness, mydriasis, visual disturbances such as yellow or green scotomata, tingling paresthesias, vertigo; initially slow pulse (less than 30) and hypotension (less than 50 mm Hg systolic), headaches, pallor, dizziness, sweating, dysphagia; then, irregular, rapid, thready pulse with blood pressure greater than 200 mm Hg; slow, shallow breathing; hypothermia, myotonia; prostration, hallucination, aphasia, syncope, hemiparesis, paralysis, confusion, hypothermia, paralysis, mild convulsions, A-V block, muscular spasms and neuropathy, sleepiness, coma; death by asphyxia rare, more often cardiac arrest.

    ECG – T wave inversion, flattening or peaking, ST depression, QT shortening.

    Chronic – Tolerance to hypotensive but not hypertensive effects develops.

Treatment:

    First Aid – Emesis if not already occurring; activated charcoal; strong tea or coffee.

    Medical – Gastric lavage with potassium permanganate solution if no emesis; tannic acid; cathartic; catheterize to stimulate elimination; atropine 0.5 mg IV for hypotension (systolic < 90mmHg) and bradycardia (pulse < 60), repeat as indicated (pressor response to atropine variable); may need metaraminol for hyptotension or sympatholytics for hypertension when due to chronic use; opium or morphine for pain and vomiting; promethazine 5 mg IV for nausea if blood pressure is stable or metoclopromide 10 mg IV for nausea and vomiting; IV diazepam for seizures. Electrolyte substitution; sodium bicarbonate for acidosis; mechanical ventilation with oxygen if necessary.

    Other – Friction rubs; recumbent with fresh air; keep horizontal, quiet, and warm. Ammonia and nux vomica. Coffee injected rectally. Demulcents for internal inflammation.

References:

1, 3, 5, 6, 7, 9, 10, 12, 14, 34, 36, 103, 104, 107, 203, 217

Veronicastrum virginicum (L.) Farw.
(= *Leptandra virginica* Nutt.)
Scrophulariaceae

Common Names:

Leptandra, black root, Culver's root, Bowman's root, tall speedwell, tall veronica, hini, oxadoddy, physic root, purple leptandra

Parts Containing Toxins:

Fresh roots and rhizomes.

Toxic Constituents – Bitter resin, cinnamic acid and para-methoxy-cinnamic acid.

Doses:

Therapeutic – Dried powder 0.65-3.89 gm; tincture 5-60 drops (0.31-3.70 ml); fluid extract 5-20 drops (0.31-1.23 ml).

Note:

Contraindications – In pregnancy it acts an an abortifacient.

Mechanism of Toxicity – The fresh root acts as a violent gastroenteric irritant.

Toxicity Signs/Symptoms:

Nausea, severe bloody diarrhea and debility.

Treatment:

(See Treatment section under Explanation of Format.)

References:

3, 9, 100

Viscum album L.;
Viscum flavescens Pursh.
(= *Phoradendron flavescens* (Pursh.) Nutt.)
Loranthaceae

Common Names:

Mistletoe, all-heal, devil's fuge, European mistletoe; American mistletoe, false mistletoe, golden bough

Parts Containing Toxins:

Leaves, top branches and berries, all parts.

Toxic Constituents – Amines of beta-phenylamine choline; viscotoxin (protein) and viscumin (glycoprotein) in *V. album* and phoratoxin (protein) in *V. flavescens*.

Doses:

Therapeutic – Powder 0.65-1.62 gm; tincture 5-60 drops (0.31-3.7 ml).

Toxic – Between 5-20 berries or 1-5 leaves may cause mild symptoms.

Lethal – Berries 1-2 in a child. Phoratoxin LD_{50} 0.57 mg/kg IP in mice.

Note:

Contraindications – In pregnancy due to the abortifacient use of *V. flavescens* by American Indians. Though it contains tyramine, a uterine stimulant in animals, the uterine activity of this constituent is unlikely with oral consumption. Avoid *V. album* parenterally in cases of protein hypersensitivity and chronic progressive infections like tuberculosis.

Mechanism of Toxicity – The viscotoxins are not absorbed orally, but may have a necrotising effect in high doses.

Other – Extracts are more potent when derived from a fresh plant.

Onset of symptoms occurs within 6 hours.

V. album is found in Europe but not America.

V. flavescens is the plants commonly sold at Christmas in the United States.

The toxicity of these parasitic species varies depending on the type of tree that they grow on.

Toxicity Signs/Symptoms:

Orally – Vomiting, bloody diarrhea, muscular spasms to the point of convulsions, prostration, mydriasis; nausea, respiratory difficulty, bradycardia, bounding pulse, profuse sweating, delirium, hallucinations, cardiovascular collapse; coma, death 10 hours after ingestion.

Parenterally – Chills, headaches, high fever, angina, circulatory disturbances, allergic reactions.

Treatment:

First Aid – Emesis; activated charcoal.

Medical – Gastric lavage if no emesis; cathartic; maintain and monitor fluid and electrolyte balance; atropine 0.6 mg IV; monitor serum potassium; for hyperkalemia hemodialysis may help restore potassium to normal, or Kayeralate (R), or glucose/insulin; for heart block use phenytoin or transvenous electrical pacemaker.

References:

3, 9, 10, 14, 25, 102, 104, 106, 107, 204

Appendix A

Potential Toxicity Of Volatile Oils Derived From Medicinal Plants

Introduction

The increasing popularity of aromatherapy has led to professional and public use of the powerful isolated essential oils of many plants. Some plants with active volatiles, such as those in list A.1, have essential oil or other components in their crude alcoholic extracts that contribute to potentially toxic activities. Other plants, including those in list A.2, are safe when used in their traditional forms as dried herbs or hydroalcoholic extracts, becasue the concentration of essential oils in fresh plants is usually in the range of only 1-2%. However, the pure volatile oil provides a concentration which might pose a potential risk. The essential oils therefore need to be considered separately in view of the dangers from using such concentrated components. This appendix addresses the need for this information.

General Considerations

Volatile oils are absorbed through the skin and mucosa. Oral use of essential oils is almost always risky due to the potential for irritation of the mucosa, whether it be gastrointestinal, rectal, or vaginal. To avoid irritation the oils should always be dispersed in a suitable carrier medium. Nausea and vomiting are common adverse effects following excessive oral doses. Toxicity is typically dose-dependent. Metabolism typically occurs in the liver where the metabolites are conjugated. Most excretion occurs via the kidneys, but some volatiles are expelled through the lungs. For certain species of plants that exist in several different chemotypes, one variety may be much higher in a toxic component than another. Isomers of the same compound can also have different toxicities.

Dose Considerations

There are a number of generalizations that can be made about essential oils that differ from crude plants or extracts. The volume of one drop of essential oil is equivalent to 0.05 ml, smaller than one minim, a standard drop of water (0.06 ml). The typical oral dosage range is from 0.5-2.5 ml/day, usually 0.5-1.0 ml/day. Cautions and contraindications, such as for oral consumption, apply for internal doses greater than 0.5 ml/day. When external applications are contraindicated, this refers to a concentration of the oil greater than 1.0% in a carrier base. Undiluted oils should not generally be used in massage nor applied to eyes, mucosa, and diseased or broken skin.

Precautions and Contraindications

For special conditions certain standards apply. In pregnancy essential oils should not be used orally, rectally, or vaginally without professional supervision, and topical applications should not exceed 2% concentration of the volatile oil. In allergies and phototoxicities even low doses can produce severe reactions. For oils with a phototoxic potential the concentration used topically should not exceed 1%, and no ultraviolet light exposure should occur for 12 hours following application to the area treated. For oils with carcinogenic potential, the maximum level for topical use should be in the range of 1.5-2.5%. Do not apply oils on or near the eyes. Do not use oils in or near the noses of children under the age of 5. Essential oils should not be used orally in children under 20 kg (45 lbs.) and should not be used topically in children under two years of age.

Treatment Of Volatile Oil Toxicities

The treatment of overdoses and poisoning with essential oil is often not specifically defined. As with other poisonings, friends or family of the victim should immediately contact a poison control center and follow the instructions given. If this is not possible or appropriate, the victim's physician or a local hospital should be contacted. Transport to the emergency room should be accomplished by the most rapid means available, preferably by ambulance so that supportive care can be provided in the interim. If possible, the source of the poison should be brought along for positive identification, and the amount ingested estimated. Because of the concentration and the rapid absorption of essential oil, rapid intervention is of utmost importance. However, emesis should not be attempted unless instructions are received to do so from medical personal, since aspirational pneumonitis may result due to the volatile irritants. Gastric lavage in a medical setting is usually the preferred means of reducing gastric absorption. In cases of topical exposure, washing the skin with soap and water may be of benefit.

Further Information

The selected plants in lists A.1 and A.2 represent sources of most of the commonly available essential oils used for their therapeutic effects, flavors and fragrance in medicine, cooking and cosmetics. For more information reference #105, *Essential Oil Safety*, edited by R. Tisserand and T. Balacs, provides in-depth discussions of these and other oils and discusses important issues regarding their safe use.

Plant Sources Of Potentially Toxic Essential Oils

A.1

PotentiallyToxic Plants

Acorus calamus, p.31
Artemisia absinthium, Artemisia spp., p.46
Brassica alba, B. juncea, B. nigra, p.55
Chenopodium ambrosioides, p.68
Cinnamomum camphora, p.73
Hedeoma pulegioides, p.112
Juniperus communis, Juniperus spp., p.124
Juniperus sabina, p.125
Mentha pulegium, p.112
Ruta graveolens, p.169
Tanacetum vulgare, p.184
Thuja occidentalis, p.188

A.2

Nontoxic Plants

Achillea millefolium, p.207
Allium cepa, A. sativa, p.208
Asarum canadense, p.209
Barosma betulina, B. crenulata , p.210
Cinnamomum cassia, C. zeylanicum , p.211
Citrus aurantium , p.212
Eucalyptus globulus, p.213
Foeniculum vulgare, p.215
Gaultheria procumbens, p.216
Hyssopus officinalis, p.218
Ledum palustre, p.218
Melaleuca alternifolia, p.219
Ocimum basilicum, p.221
Petroselinum crispum, p.222
Peumus boldus, p.223
Pimpinella anisum, p.224
Pinus palustris, P. pinaster, p.225
Piper cubeba, p. 226

Nontoxic Plant Sources Of Potentially Toxic Essential Oils

Achillea millefolium L.   Asteraceae

Common Name:

Yarrow

Parts Containing Volatile Oil:

Aerial herb 0.2-1.0%.

Toxic Constituents – Beta-isothujone or 10-20% camphor (volatile ketones) chemotypes.

Doses:

Therapeutic – Powder 1.5 gm; juice 1 tsp (3.7 ml).

Toxic – 30 mg/kg thujone.

Note:

Precautions – Avoid the use of camphor chemotype oil in epilepsy and fever.

Contraindications – In pregnancy due to its emmenagogue and abortifacient effects. Whole herb is contraindicated in allergy to yarrow and other Asteracea plants due to its sesquiterpene lactone content.

Mechanism of Toxicity – Gastrointestinal irritant and CNS stimulant.

Toxicity Signs/Symptoms:

Convulsions.

Treatment:

First Aid – Emesis or gastric lavage; activated charcoal; cathartic.

References:

2, 14, 25,100, 105, 106, 107

Allium cepa L.;
Allium sativa L.   Liliaceae

Common Names:

Onion; Garlic

Parts Containing Volatile Oil:

Bulbs, stem.

Toxic Constituents - Disulphides and trisulphides

Doses:

Therapeutic – Juice of *A. sativa* 1 tsp (3.7 ml); tincture
of *A. sativa* 5-30 drops (0.31-1.85 ml),

tincture of *A. cepa* 5-60 drops (0.31-3.7 ml).

Note:

Precautions – Use the oil orally with care in kidney and liver
disease, prostate cancer, systemic lupus erythematosis, and
with other anticoagulants such as aspirin, heparin, or
warfarin.

Contraindications – In large doses in pregnancy, since they
are reported as being emmenagogue and potentially
abortifacient, and uterine stimulation has been shown in
animals. The oils of onion and garlic should not be used
orally by people with clotting problems or thyroid disease.
Avoid external use of oil in subjects with sensitive, diseased,
or damaged skin and in children under age 2.

Mechanism of Toxicity – Garlic oil can cause local irritation
to the skin and mucosa. Garlic and its oil, especially the
component methyl allyl trisulphide, reduce platelet activity
and inhibit clotting. Allergic dermititis is caused by dially
disulphide, allicin and allylpropyl disulphide.

Other –Horses have shown primary liver and kidney damage.

Reduced iodine uptake by thyroid can be produced with a
number of *Allium* disulfides in rats. This has not been shown
in humans.

Toxicity Signs/Symptoms:

Acute – Gastroenteritis.

Lab – Leucocytosis.

Topically – *A. sativa* can cause contact dermatitis.

Treatment:

First Aid – Emesis; activated charcoal. For contact dermatitis wash exposed area twice with soap and water.

Medical – Gastric lavage if no emesis; cathartic.

References:

2, 5, 14, 25, 69, 70, 101, 105, 106, 107

Asarum canadense L.   **Aristolochiaceae**

Common Name:

Wild ginger

Parts Containing Volatile Oil:

Rhizome with 3.5-4.5%.

Toxic Constituents – 36-45% Methyleugenol and traces of beta-asarone (volatile ethers).

Doses:

Therapeutic – Powder 2-4 gm.

Lethal – Oil LD_{50} 4.48 ml/kg orally in animals; methyleugenol LD_{50} 0.81-1.56 gm/kg orally in rats.

Note:

Precautions – Avoid oral use in liver disease or alcoholism and during use of acetominophen. The rhizome should not be used long term.

Contraindications – The rhizome in pregnancy due to its emmenagogue and abortifacient effects. The essential oil should not be used internally or externally in therapy.

Mechanism of Toxicity – Methyleugenol and beta-asarone are genotoxic and carcinogenic. Methyleugenol binds to hepatic DNA and is activated to a proximate hepatic carcinogen by its conversion to a 1'-hydroxy derivative.

Other – The rhizome also contains small amounts of the nephrotoxic aristolochic acid.

The following toxicity is based on methyleugenol studies, not on *A. canadensis* oil.

Toxicity Signs/Symptoms:

[In rodents] **Chronic** - Hepatic carcinomas.

Treatment:

(See Treatment section under Appendix A, Introduction.)

References:

100, 105, 211, 212

Barosma betulina (Thunb.) Bartl. & Wendl.; *Barosma crenulata* (L.) Hook.   Rutaceae

Common Names:

Buchu; Oval buchu

Parts Containing Volatile Oil:

1.95% and 1.13%, respectively, in dried leaves.

Toxic Constituents – Isomenthone, menthone (volatile ketones) and diosphenol (volatile phenol) in *B. betulina*; pulegone, isomenthone, and isopulegone (volatile ketones) in *B. crenulata*

Doses:

Therapeutic – Powder 0.32-3.89 gm.

Note:

Precautions – Avoid oral use in liver disease or alcoholism and during use of acetominophen.

Contraindications – Leaves in pregnancy and in acute inflammation of the GU tract. The oil of *B. betulina* should not be used in pregnancy or children under 2, and

B. crenulata oil should not be used internally or externally in therapy.

Mechanism of Toxicity – Essential oils with diophenol or pulegone are irritating to mucosa. Pulegone metabolites are toxic to the liver.

Other – The leaves darken the urine with a brownish precipitate and imparts their aroma to the urine.

Toxicity Signs/Symptoms:

Gastroenteritis and strangury.

Treatment:

(See Treatment section under Appendix A, Introduction.)

References:

9, 72, 73, 100, 105, 106, 107

Cinnamomum cassia J. Presl.;
Cinnamomum zeylanicum Blume
(= *Cinnamomum verum* J.S. Presl)
Lauraceae

Common Name:

Cassia; Cinnamon

Parts Containing Volatile Oil:

Bark

Toxic Constituents – Cinnamaldehyde (volatile aldehyde); tannin.

Doses:

Therapeutic – Powder 1 gm; tincture < 4 ml; oil 0.1 ml.

Toxic – Oil 0.5 ml/kg or greater internally.

Lethal – Oil LD_{50} 2.8-3.4 mg/kg orally in animals.

Note:

Precautions – Avoid oral use in liver disease or alcoholism and during use of acetominophen.

Contraindications – In pregnancy since the bark and oil are emmenogogues and the bark is abortifacient. Avoid in individuals hypersensitive to cinnamon or Peruvian balsam. The undiluted oil should not be used internally or externally as a therapy (dilutions of 0.1% may be tolerated).

Mechanism of Toxicity – A strong local irritant in its concentrated form. Allergic reactions or sensitisation can occur in sensitive individuals.

Toxicity Signs/Symptoms:

Internal – Nausea, vomiting, burning in mouth, chest and stomach; double vision, kidney damage, collapse, coma.

External – Redness and burning, blistering; dermatitis.

Treatment:

First Aid – Emesis or gastric lavage; activated charcoal; wash thoroughly if dermal exposure.

Medical – Cathartic; maintain fluid and electrolyte balance; avoid use of drugs; obtain baseline renal and hepatic function studies.

References:

5, 6, 11, 14, 25, 105, 106, 107

Citrus aurantium L.   Rutaceae

Common Name:

Bitter orange

Parts Containing Volatile Oil:

Peel.

Toxic Constituents – 89-96% Limonene (volatile monterpene); bergapten (furanocoumarin).

Doses:

Therapeutic – Oil 0.1 ml.

Note:

Precautions – Phototoxicity can occur on exposure to ultraviolent light within 12 hours after external application of the oil

Contraindications – In gastrointestinal ulcers.

Mechanism of Toxicity – Furanocoumarins cause phototoxicity. Limonene is a mild irritant to the skin and mucosa.

Other – The expressed (not distilled) oils from the related species *Citrus bergamia* (bergamot fruit), *Citrus aurantifolia* (lime peel), *Citrus limonum* (lemon peel), and *Citrus paradisi* (grapefruit peel) also contain bergapten and can cause phototoxicity with exposure to ultravioletet within 12 hours of being applied externally.

Toxicity Signs/Symptoms:

Internal – Violent colic, convulsions, and death.

External – Dermatitis; photosensitisation.

Treatment:

First Aid – Emesis; charcoal; for dermatitis wash exposed area twice with soap and water.

Medical – Gastric lavage; cathartic.

References:

6, 14, 105, 107

Eucalyptus globulus Labill.   Myrtaceae

Common Name:

Blue gum

Parts Containing Volatile Oil:

Leaves (3-6%).

Toxic Constituents – 80-90% Eucalyptol, also called 1,8-cineole (oxide volatile oil).

Doses:

Therapeutic – Eucalyptol 1-10 drops (0.06-0.62 ml); volatile oil 1-10 drops (0.06-0.62 ml); tincture 20-60 drops (1.23-3.7 ml); fluid extract 10-60 drops (0.62-3.7 ml).

Toxic – Oil 2-10 ml in children (in some cases only a few drops), 4-30 ml in adults.

Lethal – Oil 30-60 ml.

Note:

Precaution – Should not be used by children under age 2, especially around the face and nose or by direct inhalation, since this may lead to glottal or brochial spasms.

Contraindications – In acute renal inflammations, gastrointestinal or biliary inflammation, and severe hepatic disease.

Other – Inhalation of eucalyptol increases the rate of metabolism of a number of medications.

Toxicity Signs/Symptoms:

Gastroenteritis, nausea, vomiting, diarrhea, incoordination, vertigo; depression, drowsiness, short and irregular breathing, contracted pupils; epigastric pain, weak legs, cold sweats, headache; renal congestion, muscular prostration, ataxia, collapse, hypotension; cold skin, pale lips and

cheeks, feeble pulse, coma, asphyxiation, and death.

External – Dermatitis.

Treatment:

First Aid – Activated charcoal (no emesis due to danger of aspiration).

Medical – Gastric lavage with airway protection if no spontaneous emesis. Diazepam for spasms, atropine ffor colic; monitor and replenish electrolytes; sodium bicarbonate for acidosis; mechanical ventilation with oxygen if necessary.

Other – Nux vomica, belladonna, and alcohol.

References:

3, 6, 9, 10, 59, 105, 107, 205, 208

Foeniculum vulgare (Mill.) Thellung   Apiaceae

Common Name:

Sweet fennel

Parts Containing Volatile Oil:

Seed (fruit) (2-6.5%).

Toxic Constituents – 75-92% Anethole (volatile phenolic ether), < 5% estragole (volatile ether).

Doses:

Therapeutic – Oil 0.1-0.2 ml.

Toxic – Oil 1-5 ml.

Lethal – Oil LD_{50} 3.8 gm/kg in rats.

Note:

Precaution – Do not consume the essential oil or seed extract high in anethole for more than several consecutive weeks without seeking professional advice. Avoid oral use of oil in liver disease or alcoholism, while breast-feeding, and during use of acetominophen.

Contraindications – Essesntial oil and alcoholic extracts in pregnancy due to its emmenagogue and potential abortifacient effects. Do not use essential oil for infants or toddlers.

Mechanism of Toxicity – The reactions to fennel and its oil are mostly allergic in nature. Anethole has estrogenic activity and depletes hepatic glutathione.

Toxicity Signs/Symptoms:

Skin irritation, nausea, vomiting, seizures, pulmonary edema, mild liver lesions.

External – Dermatitis.

Treatment:

(See Treatment section under Appendix A, Introduction.)

References:

5, 6, 25, 38, 100, 105, 106, 107

Gaultheria procumbens L.   **Ericaceae**

Common Name:

Wintergreen

Parts Containing Volatile Oil:

Herb.

Toxic Constituents – 98% Methyl salicylate (volatile ester).

Doses:

Therapeutic – Oil 5-15 drops (0.25-0.75ml).

Lethal – Oil 0.23-0.37 gm/kg; 4 ml oil in children (4.7 grams). LD_{50} 1.2 gm/kg orally in rodents.

Note:

Precautions – The oil should not be used in combination with anticoagulants.

Contraindications – In pregnancy due to teratogenic potential of methyl salicylate.

Kinetics – Absorbed orally and topically, distributed to most tissues, crosses the placenta and enters breast milk. Hydrolyzed by esterases in the liver and excreted in the urine (slowly if acidic).

Mechanisms of Toxicity – Methyl salicylate is a respiratory stimulant, but it uncouples mitochondrial oxidative phosphorilation and inhibits the Krebs cycle, causing mental and central depression. Renal damage occurs in overdoses.

Other – Source (synthetic or natural) should be stated on label. Almost all commercial wintergreen oil is synthetic methyl salicylate. Synthetic preparations are 99% pure, natural wintergreen oil is 98% methyl salicylate.

Sweet birch oil (*Betula lenta*) is also 98% methyl salicylate. Oil dose of 1 ml is equivalent to 1.4 grams of acetylsalicylic acid.

Toxicity Signs/Symptoms:

Acute – Respiratory stimulation (rapid and labored breathing with respiratory alkalosis), rapid heart rate, drowsiness, irritability, sweating, thirst, diarrhea, vertigo, tremors, pulmonary edema; hypertension, dizziness, tinnitus, hallucinations, garrulity, CNS disturbances (EEG), hemorrhagia, delirium, convulsions, fever, nausea and vomiting, dehydration, acidosis, encephalopathy, cardiovascular collapse, paresis, somnolence; coma and death due to respiratory failures. Death may occur after apparent recovery.

Chronic – Skin eruptions.

Lab – A 1 : 1 mixture of heated urine and 10% Fe C13 or Phenistix (R) produces a purple color. Hyperglycemia can occur in adults, whereas hypoglycemia may occur in children. Autopsy shows congestion of lungs, liver, stomach, duodenum and kidneys.

Treatment:

First Aid – Emesis; activated charcoal; treat fever with external cooling.

Medical – Gastric lavage; saline cathartic; monitor serum salicylate, electrolytes and blood gases routinely. Hospitalize immediately to see if serum levels are elevated; IV rehydration, alkalinzation; treat hypokalemia unless oliguric; hemodialysis.

References:

5, 7, 9,13, 14, 105, 107

Hyssopus officinalis L.   Lamiaceae

Common Name:

Hyssop

Parts Containing Volatile Oil:

Herb.

Toxic Constituents – 40% Pinocamphone and 30% isopinocamphone.

Doses:

Toxic – Oil 10-30 drops (0.5-1.5 ml) in adults, 2-3 drops (0.1-0.15 ml) in children.

Lethal – Oil 1.4 ml/kg orally.

Notes:

Contraindications – In pregnancy due to neurotoxic activity and emmenagogue and abortifacient effects. Do not use oil orally. Avoid using oil in children under 2 years old and in epilepsy and fever.

Mechanism of Toxicity – The oil acts as a neurotoxin similar to camphor.

Toxicity Signs/Symptoms:

Tonic-clonic spasms, convulsions.

Treatment:

(See Treatment section under Appendix A, Introduction.)

References:

105, 107

Ledum latifolium Jac.; *Ledum palustre* L.   Ericaceae

Common Name:

Labrador tea; Marsh tea

Parts Containing Volatile Oil:

Herb 0.9-2.6%.

Toxic Constituents – Ledol, also called ledum camphor (volatile sesquiterpene); leditannic acid (tannin).

Doses:

(Primarily used in homeopathic dilutions.)

Notes:

Contraindications – In pregnancy due to uterine stimulant activity and abortifacient effect of the herb and its oil.

Mechanism of Toxicity – The essential oil is a strong irritant to the skin and mucous membranes of the gastrointestinal and genitourinary tracts.

Toxicity Signs/Symptoms:

Gastroenteritis with vomiting, diarrhea, irritated kidneys, bladder and urethra; violent headache, heavy perspiration, pain in muscles and joints, excitation of central nervous system and intoxication, spasms, paralysis.

Treatment:

First Aid – Emesis; activated charcoal.

Medical – If no emesis, gastric lavage with potassium permanganate; saline cathartic; IV diazepam for spasms; atropine for colic; sodium bicarbonate for acidosis; monitor and restore electrolyte balance. Mechanical ventilation with oxygen if necessary. Monitor kidney function.

References:

25, 103, 104, 106, 107

Melaleuca alternifolia Cheel   Myrtaceae

Common Name:

Tea tree

Parts Containing Volatile Oil:

Leaves.

Toxic Constituents – Terpinen-4-ol (volatile alcohol), cineole (volatile ether).

Doses:

Toxic – Oil 10 ml in infant, in excess of 1.0 oz. (29.6 ml) in adults; orally, 0.5-1.0 ml/kg is extremely toxic.

Lethal – Oil 2 gm/kg orally in rats, LD_{50} 1.90 gm/kg orally in animals.

Notes:

Contraindications – In allergic contact dermatitis from sensitization to tea tree components, especially limonene, alpha-terpinene, aromadendrene, and eucalyptol.

Kinetics – Oil components are rapidly absorbed orally or dermally. Metabolism of terpenes occur in the liver by P-450 dependent mono-oxigenases and/or conjugation with glucuronic acid. Excretion in bile and urine in 2-3 days in rats.

Toxicity Signs/Symptoms:

Internal – Abdominal pain, diarrhea, ataxia, drowsiness, hallucinations, coma. A rash and general edema may develop in allergic sensitivities.

External – Contact dermatitis.

Treatment:

First Aid – Activated charcoal 2 gm/kg if taken orally. Wash skin in dermal exposures.

Medical – Monitor for respiratory and cardiovascular functions.

Other – check for hypothermia and give heat support as needed.

References:

105, 206, 207, 208, 209, 210

Ocimum basilicum L.   Lamiaceae

Common Name:

Basil

Parts Containing Volatile Oil:

Leaves.

Toxic Constituents – Estragole (volatile ether).

Doses:

Lethal – Oil LD_{50} 1.4 gm/kg orally in animals; estragole LD_{50} 1.25 gm/kg orally in mice.

Notes:

Precautions – Avoid oral use in liver disease or alcoholism and during use of acetominophen.

Contraindications – The leaves should not be used in large therapeutic amounts in early pregnancy. They should be avoided for young children and not used for extended periods of time. The oil should not be used internally or externally in therapy, especially in pregnancy or while nursing.

Mechanism of Toxicity – Estragole is metabolised to 1'-hydroxyestragole which is genotoxic and carcinogenic. Estragole binds to hepatic DNA where its derivative acts as a proximate carcinogen.

Other – The estragole chemotype has 40-87% estragole, while the linalool chemotype has only 1.3-16.5%. Low estragole basil has <5% and is the only that should be used therapeutically, and then only externally.

The following toxicity is based on reports on estragole, not basil oil.

Toxicity Signs/Symptoms:

Chronic – [In animals] Hepatocellular carcinoma.

Treatment:

(See Treatment section under Appendix A, Introduction.)

References:

100, 105, 107, 211, 212

Petroselinum crispum (Miller) Nyman ex A.W. Hill (= *Petroselinum sativum* (L.) Hoff.)   **Apiaceae**

Common Name:

Parsley

Parts Containing Volatile Oil:

Seed (fruit) 0.05-0.12%.

Toxic Constituents – Apiol, myristicin (volatile phenolic ethers).

Doses:

Therapeutic – Powder 1 gm; oil 0.3-1 ml; apiol 200-500 mg.

Toxic – Oil 6 grams (in 48 hours); apiol 2-4 gm.

Lethal – Oil LD_{50} 1.52 gm/kg orally in mice, 3.96 gm/kg orally in rats; apiol 4.2 gm.

Note:

Precautions – Do not combine seed oil with meperidine (pethidine) due to the monoamine oxidase inhibition of the major oil component myristicin.

Contraindications – The oils of the leaf and seed and alcoholic extracts of the seed should be avoided in pregnancy due to its emmenagogue and abortifacient effects and uterine stimulant activity in animals. Avoid in patients with allergy to apiol and those with kidney inflammation. Do not rely on diuretic effects ofr edema from reduced cardiac or kidney function.

Mechanism of Toxicity – Vascular congestion and increased contractility of smooth muscle of bladder, intestines, and especially uterus are produced by the oil and apiol. Severe renal damage occurs due to the apiol. The oil is a mucosal irritant.

Other – The risk from aqueous extracts is less due to the lower essential oil content.

Contact dermatitis and photodermatosis are possible due to berapten and other furanocoumarins.

Typical commercial oil has 21% apiol, 28% myristicin and 23% tetramethoxyallylbenzene. The three chemotypes of parsley based on these three major compounds have apiol contents of 58-80%, 0-3%, and 0-trace.

Toxicity Signs/Symptoms:

Increased sense of bodily warmth, vertigo, headache, tinnitus, visual disturbances, scintillation; nausea, vomiting, emaciation; urticaria, swollen or fatty liver and mild icterus; irritation and mucosal bleeding from GI and GU tracts, renal epithelial damage, anuria; cardiac arrhythmias.

Treatment:

(See Treatment section under Appendix A, Introduction.)

References:

3, 5, 9, 25, 100, 104, 105, 106, 107

Peumus boldus Molina   Monimiaceae

Common Name:

Boldo

Parts Containing Volatile Oil:

Dried leaves.

Toxic Constituents – 16-40% Ascaridole (volatile terpene).

Doses:

Therapeutic – Powder 1.5 gm.

Toxic – Oil LD_{50} 0.07 gm/kg orally in rats.

Lethal – Oil LD_{50} 0.13 gm/kg orally in animals.

Note:

Precautions – Patients with gallstones should consult physician before use.

Contraindications – The leaves should be avoided in bile duct obstruction and severe liver diseases. The oil should not be used therapeutically either internally or externally.

Mechanism of Toxicity – The volatile oil is strongly neurotoxic.

Toxicity Signs/Symptoms:

Convulsions, paralysis.

Treatment:

(See Treatment section under Appendix A, Introduction.)

References:

105, 107

Pimpinella anisum L.   Apiaceae

Common Name:

Anise

Parts Containing Volatile Oil:

Seed (fruit) (1-3%).

Toxic Constituents – 80-90% Anethole (volatile phenolic ether), <4% estragole (volatile ether).

Doses:

Therapeutic – Oil 0.2-0.3 ml.

Toxic – Oil 1-5 ml.

Lethal – Oil LD_{50} 2.25 gm/kg orally in animals;

anethole 2.1 gm/kg in rats.

Note:

Precautions – Avoid oral use of oil in liver disease or alcoholism, while breast-feeding, and during use of acetominophen.

Contraindications – In pregnancy (including whole seed or fruit) and in allergies to anise or anethole.

Mechanism of Toxicity – Reactions mostly due to allergic response. Anethole has estrogenic effects and depletes glutathione in liver cells.

Toxicity Signs/Symptoms:

Skin irritation, nausea, vomiting, seizures or pulmonary edema, mild liver lesions.

Treatment:

(See Treatment section under Appendix A, Introduction.)

References:

5, 38, 100, 105, 106, 107

Pinus palustris Mill.
(= *Pinus australis* Michaux fililus),
Pinus pinaster Aiton   Pinaceae

Common Name:

Gum turpentine tree

Parts Containing Volatile Oil:

Wood oleoresin .

Toxic Constituents – 50-64% Alpha-pinene, 25-35% beta-pinene, and 20-60% delta-3-carene (volatile monoterpenes).

Doses:

Therapeutic – Rectified turpentine oil 1-10 drops (0.05-0.5ml).

Note:

Precautions – Only rectified oil of turpentine is used medicinally.

Topical application to extensive surface areas can cause symptoms of poisoning.

Contraindications – In pregnancy due to its abortifacient effect and in acute nephritis. Avoid where there is a hypersensitivity to essential oils. Do not use as inhalation therapy for acute respiratory tract inflammation.

Mechanism of Toxicity – The oil turpentine acts as a local irritant.

Other – An odor of violets is imparted to the urine.

Toxicity Signs/Symptoms:

Internal – Burning pain in the stomach, nausea and vomiting, eructations, diarrhea, hypertension, irritation to the GI and breathing passages; intoxication, vertigo, dizziness; irritation and hyperemia of the kidneys, albuminuria, hematuria; strangury, priapism, aching in the loins, acute glomerulonephritis, cyanosis, dilated pupils, gastroenteritis, collapse, vesicular or papular rashes of an eczematous type; abortions, hypertension, hyperpyrexia, loss of strength, trembling, incoordination, nervous irritation, wandering mind, incoherence, coma, labored breathing, paralysis of respiration; face cyanotic or flushed, pupils dilated, death.

External – Irritation and reddening; vesiculation and ulceration if contact prolonged or hot (for example, friction); damage to kidneys and central nervous system.

Treatment:

(See Treatment section under Appendix A, Introduction.)

References:

3, 6, 9, 10, 105, 106

Piper cubeba L. fil.   Piperaceae

Common Name:

Cubeb

Parts Containing Volatile Oil:

Unripe fruit.

Toxic Constituents – 1-3.5% Cubebic acid and a volatile sequiterpene.

Doses:

Therapeutic – Powder 0.2-1.6 gm; fluid extract 5-30 drops (0.3-1.9 ml); oil 1-15 drops (0.05-0.75 ml).

Toxic – Powder > 8 gm.

Note:

Mechanism of Toxicity – The oil acts as a local irritant.

Toxicity Signs/Symptoms:

Urinary tract irritation, kidney and bladder pains; nausea, vomiting, diarrhea, burning pains, fever, cardiac pains, drug dermatitis.

Lab – Albuminuria.

Treatment:

First Aid – Emesis.

Medical – Gastric lavage if no emesis; saline cathartic.

Other – Treat symptomatically.

References:

3, 5, 9, 10, 107

Rosmarinus officinalis L.   Lamiaceae

Common Name:

Rosemary

Parts Containing Volatile Oil: Leaves 1.0-2.5%.

Toxic Constituents – 10-25% camphor (volatile ketone), 10-27% alpha-pinene, 17-50% (volatile terpene), 1,8-cineole (volatile oxide).

Doses:

Therapeutic – Powder 1.3-2.0 gm.

Lethal – Oil LD_{50} 5.0 ml/kg orally in animals.

Note:

Precautions – Use carefully in fevers and epilepsy due to camphor inducing epileptiform convulsions.

Contraindications – In pregnancy due to camphor content.

Other – Tunisian oil has a lower camphor content and is probably safer.

Toxicity Signs/Symptoms:

Vomiting, gastroenteritis, spasms, uterine bleeding, kidney irritation, coma, and pulmonary edema leading to death.

Treatment:

(See Treatment section under Appendix A, Introduction.)

References:

105, 107

Salvia officinalis L.   Lamiaceae

Common Name:

Sage

Parts Containing Volatile Oil:

Leaves with 1.0-3.5%.

Toxic Constituents – 20-60% Alpha- and beta-thujone, 14-37% camphor (volatile ketones), cineole (volatile oxide).

Doses:

Therapeutic – Powder 1.3-4 grams; tincture 0.8-2.5 ml; essential oil 0.03-0.1 gm.

Toxic – Powder 15 gm; oil 0.5 gm/kg in rats;

thujone 30 mg/kg body weight.

Lethal – Oil LD_{50} 2.6 gm/kg orally in animals;

thujone LD_{50} 0.21 gm/kg orally in rodents.

Note:

Contraindications – The alcoholic extract should not be used in pregnancy, since its emmenagogue action may produce an abortion. The essential oil should not be used internally or externally in pregnancy or for therapy.

Toxicity Signs/Symptoms:

Dry mouth, local irritation, sense of heat, rapid heart rate, dizziness, epileptiform convulsions.

Treatment:

(See Treatment section under Appendix A, Introduction.)

References:

2, 5, 11, 25, 100, 101, 105, 106

Sassafras albidum (Nutt.) Nees   Lauraceae

Common Name:

Sassafras

Parts Containing Volatile Oil:

Root with about 2% oil or bark of root 6-9%.

Toxic Constituents – 85-90% Safrole (volatile phenolic ether).

Doses:

Therapeutic – Root bark extract 2.0-4.0 ml.

Toxic – Powder 100 grams; oil 4-60 ml; safrole 650 mg/kg orally in rats for 4 days.

Lethal – Oil LD_{50} 1.52-2.37 gm/kg in rats; safrole LD_{50} 1.95 and 2.35 gm/kg acutely in rats and mice, respectively; 750 mg/kg orally in rats for 19 days.

Note:

Precautions – Avoid oral use in liver disease or alcoholism and during use of acetominophen. Do not use long term.

Contraindications – The root in pregnancy due to its reported emmenagogue effect. The oil should not be used internally or externally in therapy.

Kinetics – Safrole is rapidly absorbed, and more than 90% is excreted in 24 hours. The major metabolite in humans is 4-allylcatecyol.

Mechanism of Toxicity – Safrole and sassafras oil can cause kidney damage in acute overdose. Oil of sassafras containing safrole is potentially a hepatic carcinogen when injected or consumed over long periods by animals. The safrole metabolite 1'-hydroxysafrole is an even more potent carcinogen. Both bind to hepatic DNA. These compounds may activate a cancer-causing virus in rats. Carcinogenesis was also noted in rats by injecting a safrole-free extract of *S. albidum* subcutaneously.

Other – Safrole is a potent inhibitor of liver microsomal hydroxylating systems, which may block the metabolism of certain toxic drugs.

Toxicity Signs/Symptoms:

Acute – Nausea, vomiting, dilated pupils, tachycardia, tremors, cardiovascular collapse, CNS depression; hallucinations, intermittent unconsciousness; respiratory paralysis, fatty degeneration of heart, liver and kidneys; stupor, ataxia, ptosis, hypersensitivity to touch, hypothermia.

Chronic – Cumulative effects may occur such as hepatomas, lymphomas, pulmonary adenomas, and adenocarcinomas in infant male mice given safrole.

External – Dermatitis.

Treatment:

First Aid – Emesis; activated charcoal.

Medical – Gastric lavage; cathartic; establish respiration, with respirator if necessary; obtain baseline hepatic function studies.

References:

5, 6, 14, 21, 23, 102, 105, 107, 211, 212

Syzygium aromaticum (L.) Merr. & L.M. Perry
(= *Caryophyllus aromaticus* L.)
(= *Eugenia caryophyllata* Thunb.)
Myrtaceae

Common Name:

Cloves

Parts Containing Volatile Oils:

14% Dried flowering buds.

Toxic Constituents – 70-95% Eugenol (volatile phenol).

Doses:

Toxic – Oil 5-10 ml in young children (0.3-0.7 ml/kg of eugenol).

Lethal – Oil LD_{50} 2.65 gm/kg orally in animals.

Note:

Precautions – Avoid using in alcoholism, hemophilia, kidney disease, liver disease, prostatic cancer or systemic lupus erythematosis. Do not combine with acetominophen or anticoagulants such as aspirin, heparin or warfarin. Do not use topically on children under age 2 or where there is diseased or damaged skin or hypersensitivity. Do not apply undiluted to skin.

Mechanism of Toxicity – The aromatic oil is an irritant to the mucosa. Eugenol is hepatotoxic and inhibits blood clotting.

Toxicity Signs/Symptoms:

Internal – Gastroenteritis, CNS depression, seizures, coma.

Lab – Acidosis; ketones in urine; hypoglycemia.

External – Dermatitis.

Treatment:

(See Treatment section under Appendix A, Introduction.)

References:

3, 6, 105, 106, 107

Thymus serpyllum L.;
Thymus vulgaris L.   **Lamiaceae**

Common Names:

Mother of thyme; thyme

Parts Containing Volatile Oil:

Leaves.

Toxic Constituents – Thymol, carvacrol (volatile phenols).

(The thymol and carvacrol contents vary respectively in the following T. vulgaris chemotypes with oil yields of 1.0-2.5%: thymol chemotype 32-63% and 1-5%, carvacrol chemotype 1-13% and 23-44%, thymol/carvacrol chemotype 26% and 26%. T. serpyllum yields 0.2-0.6% oil with 1-16% thymol and 21-37% carvacrol.)

Doses:

Therapeutic – Powder 1.3-2.0 gm; thymol 125 mg.

Toxic – Oil 0.2-1 ml; thymol 1-5 grams.

Lethal – Oil LD_{50} 4.7 gm/kg orally in animals.

Note:

Precautions – Use topically, including baths, with care for individuals who have hypersensitive, diseased or damaged skin, cardiac insufficiency or hypertonia, severe fevers, or for children under age 2.

Contraindications – The emmenagogue activity of *T. vulgaris* plant makes it a potential abortifacient in early pregnancy, while *T. serpyllum* has shown emmenagogue and abortifacient effects.

Mechanism of Toxicity – The oil is a strong mucous membrane irritant.

Toxicity Signs/Symptoms:

Internal – Warmth in stomach, diarrhea, nephritis with albuminuria and hematuria; profuse sweating, reduced temperature.

External – Dermatitis.

Treatment:

First Aid – Dilute with water or milk immediately; activated charcoal; emesis if less than 5% solution ingested.

Medical – Gastric lavage if greater than 5% solution ingested; saline cathartic or castor oil (30-60 ml); obtain baseline liver and renal measurements; monitor acid/base balance closely; monitor cardiac function closely; IV diazepam for seizures; 0.2 mg/kg IV methylene blue for methemoglobinemia; lidocaine for cardiac arrythmias.

References:

3, 5, 6, 9, 11, 14, 25, 105, 107

Appendix B

Botanical Medicines That May Disrupt Pregnancy

Introduction

Any herb considered potentially toxic must be appreciated as being more so in pregnancy when the developing fetus is highly susceptible to disrupting influences. These herbs must be used only when necessary and in doses well below the therapeutic maximum. Any plant used in a form that is potentially toxic is best avoided, and therefore contraindicated, during pregnancy. This includes essential oils which have a strong risk of fetotoxicity in even relatively small doses.

Potentially disruptive plants listed below exert an influence that is directly threatening to a normal pregnancy, either by upsetting the fetal development or by inducing uterine contractions. These herbs must be avoided, especially in the first trimester if they are emmenagogues, throughout pregnancy if they are teratogenic, and before the ninth month if they are certain uterine stimulants. After this time, some uterine tonic herbs may be safe when appropriately applied in the proper dosage to prepare the uterus for labor or to treat problems unrelated to pregnancy. As should be obvious, the higher the dose, the more likely that adverse effects will occur.

Essential Oils And Other Forms

The essential oils of certain nontoxic plants can act as potent uterine stimulants. When used as a crude herb or water extract, their volatile oils are unlikely to have this effect due to the reduced quantity of the volatile components consumed. This includes their use as culinary seasonings or mildly flavored beverage teas. Large and/or frequent doses of alcoholic extracts of these plants will provide significant amounts of the volatiles, and may be a risk during pregnancy. These extracts should only be used under the supervision of a qualified practitioner. The use of essential oils internally (orally, rectally, or vaginally) should be avoided in pregnancy, and broad topical applications (e.g., in massage oils) should be used in concentrations of less than 2%. Some plants that have toxic and/or uterine stimulant essential oils contain other uterine stimulant components found in active amounts in their aqueous or hydroalcoholic extracts. These plants need to be avoided in all of these forms. Such herbs will appear both in list B.1b for potentially toxic essential oils from nontoxic plants and list B.2 for nontoxic plants.

Uterotropic Effects

Nontoxic plants listed are threatening due to their uterine stimulant activity only when used during pregnancy. When these herbs are used in potent medicinal doses, the effects are more certain, being dose dependent. It is important to note the part of the plant that is contraindicated; the medicinal portion may be different than the part normally consumed as a dietary or beverage item. The terminology for those herbs that are listed in B.2 is taken from a literature review by Farnsworth et al., (reference 25) of uterine active plants based on both folkloric use and scientific research. When this reference appears in the main body of this text, the same meaning is intended for the following terms: emmenagogue, oxytocic, (possible or human) abortifacient, uterine stimulant, and isolated uterine stimulant.

Some of the herbs have been identified in folklore as emmenagogues that stimulate the onset of menses. (Emmenagogues are not always abortifacients but are contraindicated in early pregnancy. Under professional or expert care some herbs identified as emmenagogues may be used with caution in later pregnancy in small amounts as tonics). Oxytocics are uterine stimulants that have been used to strengthen contractions during labor. The herbs reported to have caused miscarriages in humans are termed human abortifacients. Plants producing abortions in animals (usually in very large quantities) are identified as potential abortifacients. Some herbs have been shown to produce uterine stimulant effects on living animals (*in vivo*) or on their isolated organs (*in vitro*). Where an isolated constituent has been shown to be a uterine stimulant, it is also listed.

Qualifying Considerations

The following lists can not be considered complete, since the emphasis is on those herbs commonly utilized in America. Not all herbs containing substances potentially toxic to the fetus (for instance, as identified through animal testing by injection of isolated constituents) have been included here, if there is no documented evidence of actual adverse effects resulting from oral consumption of the herbs. Medicinal use of any herb during pregnancy should only be done under supervision of a doctor or practitioner familiar with the pharmacological effect of the herb and well-informed regarding its influence on the physiology of pregnancy.

These lists are especially pertinent when the herbs are used in large medicinal doses. This particularly applies to the plants listed as nontoxic that may be used occasionally in small amounts. However, the medicinal application or consumption of volatile oils from nontoxic plants should generally be avoided due to the extreme concentration of active components. External application of certain volatile oils locally, or over larger areas of skin when diluted in oil for massage by knowledgeable practitioners, may be appropriate.

B.1
Potentially Toxic Herbs & Essential Oils Contraindicated in Pregnancy

B.1a
Potentially Toxic Herbs

B.1b

Potentially Toxic Essential Oils from Nontoxic Plants

B.2
Nontoxic Herbs Contraindicated in Pregnancy in Large Doses

Uterotropic Plants

Hyssopus officinalis, p.251

Jateorhiza palmata, p.251

Lavandula officinalis #, p.252

Leonurus cardiaca, p.252

Levisticum officinale, p.252

Ligusticum porteri, p.252

Marrubium vulgare, p.253

Matricaria chamomile #, p.253

Melissa officinalis #, p.253

Mentha x piperita #, p.253

Monarda spp., p.254

Nardostachys jatamansi, p.254

Nasturtium officinale, p.254

Nepeta cataria, p.254

Ocimum basilicum #, p.255

Origanum marjorana #, p.255

Origanum vulgare, p.255

Oxalis acetosella #, p.255

Paeonia officinalis, p.256

Piper nigrum, p.256

Polygonum aviculare, p.256

Rosmarinus officinalis, p.256

Rubia tinctorum, p.257

Santalum album, p.257

Silybum marianum #, p.257

Tanacetum parthenium #, p.257

Trichosanthes kirilowii, p.258

Trigonella foenumgraecum, p.258

Trillium erectum, p.258

Urtica dioica, U. urens, p.258

Verbena hastata, V. officinalis, p.259

Vetiveria zizanoides, p.259

Vitex agnus-castus, p.259

Withania somnifera, p.259

Zanthoxylum spp., p.260

Zingiber officinale, p.260

Ziziphus spp., p.260

Note:

* Contraindicated even at normal doses.

 # Contraindicated primarily in early pregnancy.

Nontoxic Herbs Contraindicated in Pregnancy in Large Doses

Agave americana L.   Agavaceae

Common Name: Agave
Parts Contraindications: Whole plant, juice, leaf juice
Uterotropic Constituents: (Not identified.)
Described Activity: Emmenagogue, abortifacient.
References: 25

Angelica archangelica L.;
Angelica atropurpurea L.;
Angelica sylvestris L.   Apiaceae

Common Names: Angelica; American angelica; European wild angelica
Parts Contraindications: Whole plant; root, seed; root
Uterotropic Constituents: (Not identified.)
Described Activity: Emmenagogue.
References: 25, 100, 104

Apium graveolens L.   Apiaceae

Common Name: Celery
Parts Contraindications: Root, fruit (seeds).
Uterotropic Constituents: Volatile oil with apiol.
Described Activity: Uterine stimulant, abortifacient.
References: 25, 100, 104, 105

Arctium lappa L.   Asteraceae

Common Name: Burdock
Parts Contraindications: (Not identified.)
Uterotropic Constituents: (Not identified.)

Described Activity: Uterine stimulant.
References: 25

Arctostaphylos uva-ursi (L.) Spreng.   Ericaceae

Common Name: Bearberry
Parts Contraindications: Leaves.
Uterotropic Constituents: (Not identified.)
Described Activity: Oxytocic.
References: 11, 100, 106, 107

Armoracia spp.   Brassicaceae

Common Name: Horseradish
Parts Contraindications: Root
Uterotropic Constituents: (Not identified.)
Described Activity: Abortifacient.
References: 104

Artemisia douglasiana Bess., *Artemisia lactiflora* Wall. ex DC., *Artemisia vulgaris* L.   Asteraceae

Common Name: Mugwort
Parts Contraindications: Whole plant, leaves, flower, roots.
Uterotropic Constituents: Thujone
Described Activity: Uterine stimulant, emmenagogue, abortifacient.
References: 25, 85, 100

Asarum canadense L.   Aristolochiaceae

Common Name: Wild ginger
Parts Contraindications: Rhizome.

Uterotropic Constituents: (Not identified.)
Described Activity: Emmenagogue.
References: 100

Beta vulgaris L.   Chenopodiaceae

Common Name: Beet
Parts Contraindications: Seed, root, leaves.
Uterotropic Constituents: (Not identified.)
Described Activity: Emmenagogue, abortifacient.
References: 25

Brayera anthelmintica Kunt
(= *Hagenia abyssinica* (Bruce) Gmelin)
Rosaceae

Common Name: Kousso
Parts Contraindications: Fresh female inflorescence.
Uterotropic Constituents: Brayerin (resin); cosotoxin.
Described Activity: Abortifacient due to irritation to the
gastrointestinal tract.
References: 10

Calendula officinalis L.   Asteraceae

Common Name: Pot marigold
Parts Contraindications: Whole plant, flowers.
Uterotropic Constituents: (Not identified.)
Described Activity: Emmenagogue, abortifacient.
References: 25

Capsella bursa-pastoris (L.) Medik.   **Brassicaceae**

Common Name: Shepherd's purse

Parts Contraindications: Whole plant, root.

Uterotropic Constituents: Tyramine. [The uterine activity of tyramine is unlikely with oral use.]

Described Activity: Isolated uterine stimulant, emmenagogue, abortifacient.

References: 25, 100, 104, 107

Carica papaya L.   **Caricaceae**

Common Name: Papaya

Parts Contraindications: Latex, fruit, seed.

Uterotropic Constituents: 5-hydroxytryptamine.

Described Activity: Isolated uterine stimulant, emmenagogue, abortifacient.

References: 25, 107

Carthamus tinctorius L.   **Asteraceae**

Common Name: Safflower

Parts Contraindications: Flower.

Uterotropic Constituents: [Not indicated

Described Activity: Emmenagogue, abortifacient.

References: 100, 107

Centella asiatica (L.) Urban.
(= *Hydrocotyle asiatica* L.)   **Apiaceae**

Common Name: Gotu kola

Parts Contraindications: Plant.

Uterotropic Constituents: (Not identified.)

Described Activity: Abortifacient.

References: 25

Chamaelirium luteum (L.) A. Gray.   Liliaceae

Common Name: Helonias
Parts Contraindications: Rhizome.
Uterotropic Constituents: [Not indicated.]
Described Activity: Emmenagogue.
References: 100

Chamaemelum nobile (L.) All.
(= *Anthemis nobilis* L.)   Asteraceae

Common Name: Roman chamomile
Parts Contraindications: Flower, whole plant.
Uterotropic Constituents: Volatile oil
Described Activity: Emmenagogue, abortifacient.
References: 25, 100

Cichorium intybus L.   Asteraceae

Common Name: Chicory
Parts Contraindications: Whole plant, seed, root.
Uterotropic Constituents: (Not identified.)
Described Activity: Emmenagogue, abortifacient.
References: 25, 104

Cinnamomum cassia J. Presl.;
Cinnamomum zeylanicum Blume
(= *Cinnamomum verum J.S. Presl)*
Lauraceae

Common Names: Cassia; Cinnamon
Parts Contraindications: Bark.
Uterotropic Constituents: (Not identified.)

Described Activity: Emmenagogue, abortifacient
References: 25, 100, 106, 107

Citrus spp.   Rutaceae

Common Names: Lemon, grapefruit, etc.

Parts Contraindications: (Not identified.) [Activity only described for the isolated constituents.]

Uterotropic Constituents: Hesperidin, tyramine. [Uterine activity of oral tyramine unlikely.]

Described Activity: Isolated uterine stimulant.

References: 25

Commiphora molmol Engl. ex Tschirsh, *Commiphora myrrha* (Nees) Engl.; *Commiphora mukul* (Hook. ex Stocks) Engl.
Burseraceae

Common Name: Myrrh; Guggul

Parts Contraindications: Gum resin.

Uterotropic Constituents: (Not identified.)

Described Activity: Emmenagogue, abortifacient.

References: 25, 100

Coptis chinensis Franch.; *Coptis groenlandica* (Oed.) Fern.   Ranunculaceae

Common Names: Chinese goldthread; Goldthread

Parts Contraindications: Rhizome.

Uterotropic Constituents: Berberine

Described Activity: Emmenagogue.

References: 100

Curcuma aromatica Salisbury.,
Curcuma domestica Valet.,
Curcuma longa L. Zingiberaceae

Common Name: Turmeric

Parts Contraindications: Rhizome.

Uterotropic Constituents: (Not identified.)

Described Activity: Uterine stimulant, emmenagogue, abortifacient.

References: 25, 100

Curcuma zedoaria (Berg.) Roscoe. Zingiberaceae

Common Name: Zedoary

Parts Contraindications: Rhizome.

Uterotropic Constituents: (Not identified.)

Described Activity: Abortifacient.

References: 25, 100

Cymbopogon citratus (DC. ex Nees) Stapf.
Poaceae

Common Name: Lemongrass

Parts Contraindications: Plant.

Uterotropic Constituents: (Not identified.)

Described Activity: Uterine stimulant, emmenagogue.

References: 25, 100

Daucus carota L. Apiaceae

Common Name: Queen Ann's lace

Parts Contraindications: Seed (fruit), leaves, root.

Uterotropic Constituents: (Not identified.)

Described Activity: Uterine stimulant, emmenagogue, abortifacient.

References: 25, 100

Ferula assa-foetida L.,
Ferula foetida (Bunge) Regel.,
Ferula rubricaulis Boiss.   **Apiaceae**

Common Name: Asafetida
Parts Contraindications: Roots and rhizomes
Uterotropic Constituents: Oleo gum-resin
Described Activity: Emmenagogue, abortifacient.
References: 25, 100

Gossypium herbaceum L.;
Gossypium hirsutum L.   **Malvaceae**

Common Names: Levant cotton; cotton
Parts Contraindications: Root bark, seeds, whole plant.
Uterotropic Constituents: (Not identified.)
Described Activity: Emmenagogue, oxytocic, abortifacient.
References: 25, 100, 104, 107

Heracleum lanatum Michx.   **Apiaceae**

Common Name: Cow parsnip
Parts Contraindications: Whole plant.
Uterotropic Constituents: (Not identified.)
Described Activity: Emmenagogue.
References: 11

Hibiscus rosa-sinensis   **Malvaceae**

Common Name: Rose of China
Parts Contraindications: Flowers.
Uterotropic Constituents: (Not identified.)
Described Activity: Emmenagogue, abortifacient.
References: 25, 104

Hypericum perforatum L.   **Hypericaceae**

Common Name: St. John's wort
Parts Contraindications: Leaves, whole plant.
Uterotropic Constituents: (Not identified.)
Described Activity: Uterine stimulant, emmenagogue,
    abortifacient.
References: 25

Hyssopus officinalis L.   **Lamiaceae**

Common Name: Hyssop
Parts Contraindications: Leaves, plant.
Uterotropic Constituents: (Not identified.)
Described Activity: Emmenagogue, abortifacient.
References: 25, 100, 104

Jateorhiza palmata (Lam.) Miers
(= *Cocculus palmatus* Wall.)   **Ranunculaceae**

Common Name: Columba
Parts Contraindications: (Not identified.) [Activity has only been
    described for the isolated constituent.]
Uterotropic Constituents: Palmitine.
Described Activity: Isolated uterine stimulant.
References: 25

Lavandula angustifolia Mill.
(= *Lavandula officinalis* Chaich.)
(= *Lavavandula vera* DC.)   Lamiaceae

Common Name: Lavender
Parts Contraindications: Flowers
Uterotropic Constituents: Coumarin
Described Activity: Emmenagogue
References: 11

Leonurus cardiaca L.   Lamiaceae

Common Name: Motherwort
Parts Contraindications: Plant.
Uterotropic Constituents: Stachydrine, leonurine.
Described Activity: Isolated uterine stimulants, emmenagogue.
References: 25, 100, 104

Levisticum officinale W. Koch.   Apiaceae

Common Name: Lovage
Parts Contraindications: Root.
Uterotropic Constituents: [Not indicated.]
Described Activity: Emmenagogue.
References: 100, 104

Ligusticum porteri J.M. Coulter & J.M. Rose
Apiaceae

Common Name: Osha
Parts Contraindications: Root.
Uterotropic Constituents: [Not indicated.]

Described Activity: Emmenagogue, abortifacient
References: 100, 115

Marrubium vulgare L.   **Lamiaceae**

Common Name: Horehound
Parts Contraindications: Whole plant.
Uterotropic Constituents: (Not identified.)
Described Activity: Uterine stimulant, emmenagogue,
   abortifacient.
References: 25, 100

Matricaria recutita L.
(= *Matricaria chamomilla* L.)   **Asteraceae**

Common Name: German chamomile
Parts Contraindications: Whole plant.
Uterotropic Constituents: (Not identified.)
Described Activity: Emmenagogue.
References: 25

Melissa officinalis L.   **Lamianceae**

Common Name: Lemon balm
Parts Contraindications: Leaves, flowers.
Uterotropic Constituents: (Not identified.)
Described Activity: Emmenagogue.
References: 25, 104

Mentha x piperita L.   **Lamiaceae**

Common Name: Peppermint
Parts Contraindications: Leaves, flowers.
Uterotropic Constituents: (Not identified.)

Described Activity: Emmenagogue.
References: 25

Monarda spp.   Lamiaceae

Common Name: Beebalm
Parts Contraindications: Plant.
Uterotropic Constituents: (Not identified.)
Described Activity: Emmenagogue.
References: 100, 107

Nardostachys jatamansi (D. Don) DC.
Valerianaceae

Common Name: Nard
Parts Contraindications: Root, rhizome.
Uterotropic Constituents: (Not identified.)
Described Activity: Emmenagogue, abortifacient.
References: 25, 100

Nasturtium officinale R. Br.   Brassicaceae

Common Name: Watercress
Parts Contraindications: Whole plant, leaf.
Uterotropic Constituents: (Not identified.)
Described Activity: Emmenagogue, abortifacient.
References: 25, 100

Nepeta cataria L.   Lamiaceae

Common Name: Catnip
Parts Contraindications: Whole plant, leaves, flowers.
Uterotropic Constituents: (Not identified.)

Described Activity: Emmenagogue, abortifacient.
References: 25, 100

Ocimum basilicum L.   **Lamiaceae**

Common Name: Basil
Parts Contraindications: Whole plant.
Uterotropic Constituents: (Not identified.)
Described Activity: Emmenagogue, abortifacient.
References: 11, 25, 100, 106, 107

Origanum marjorana L.
(= *Majorana hortensis* Moench.)   **Lamiaceae**

Common Name: Sweet marjoram
Parts Contraindications: Whole plant.
Uterotropic Constituents: (Not identified.)
Described Activity: Emmenagogue.
References: 11

Origanum vulgare L.   **Lamiaceae**

Common Name: Wild marjoram
Parts Contraindications: Whole plant.
Uterotropic Constituents: (Not identified.)
Described Activity: Emmenagogue, abortifacient.
References: 25

Oxalis acetosella L.   **Oxalidaceae**

Common Name: Wood sorrel
Parts Contraindications: Whole plant.
Uterotropic Constituents: (Not identified.)
Described Activity: Emmenagogue.
References: 2

Paeonia officinalis L.   **Paeoniaceae**

Common Name: Peony
Parts Contraindications: Root.
Uterotropic Constituents: (Not identified.)
Described Activity: Emmenagogue, abortifacient.
References: 25, 107

Piper nigrum L.   **Piperaceae**

Common Name: Black pepper
Parts Contraindications: Fruit.
Uterotropic Constituents: (Not identified.)
Described Activity: Abortifacient.
References: 25

Polygonum aviculare L.   **Polygonaceae**

Common Name: Knot grass
Parts Contraindications: (Not identified.)
Uterotropic Constituents: (Not identified.)
Described Activity: Human abortifacient.
References: 25

Rosmarinus officinalis L.   **Lamiaceae**

Common Name: Rosemary
Parts Contraindications: Flowers, leaves.
Uterotropic Constituents: Camphor.
Described Activity: Emmenagogue, abortifacient.
References: 25, 100, 104, 105, 107

Rubia tinctorum L.   Rubiaceae

Common Name: Madder
Parts Contraindications: Root.
Uterotropic Constituents: [Not indicated.]
Described Activity: Emmenagogue.
References: 101, 104

Santalum album L.   Santalaceae

Common Name: Sandalwood
Parts Contraindications: (Not identified.)
Uterotropic Constituents: (Not identified.)
Described Activity: Abortifacient.
References: 25

Silybum marianum (L.) Gaertn.   Asteraceae

Common Name: Milk thistle
Parts Contraindications: Root, herb, seed.
Uterotropic Constituents: Tyramine. [The uterine activity of tyramine is unlikely with oral use.]
Described Activity: Isolated uterine stimulant, emmenagogue.
References: 25, 107

Tanacetum parthenium (L.) Schultz-Bip.
     Asteraceae

Common Name: Feverfew
Parts Contraindications: Whole plant.
Uterotropic Constituents: (Not identified.)
Described Activity: Emmenagogue.
References: 25, 100

Trichosanthes kirilowii Maxim.   Cucurbitaceae

Common Name: Chinese cucumber
Parts Contraindications: Root.
Uterotropic Constituents: (Not identified.)
Described Activity: Abortifacient.
References: 100

Trigonella foenum-graecum L.   Fabaceae

Common Name: Fenugreek
Parts Contraindications: Seed, whole plant.
Uterotropic Constituents: (Not identified.)
Described Activity: Uterine stimulant, emmenagogue, abortifacient.
References: 25, 100

Trillium erectum L.
(= *Trillium pendulum* Muhl.)   Liliaceae

Common Name: Birth root
Parts Contraindications: Root.
Uterotropic Constituents: (Not identified.)
Described Activity: Emmenagogue, oxytocic.
References: 100, 104, 107

Urtica dioica L.;
Urtica urens L.   Urticaceae

Common Names: Stinging nettle; dwarf nettle
Parts Contraindications: Whole plant.
Uterotropic Constituents: 5-hydroxytryptamine.
Described Activity: Isolated uterine stimulant, emmenagogue, abortifacient.
References: 25

Verbena hastata L.;
Verbena officinalis L. Verbenaceae

Common Names: Blue vervain; European vervain
Parts Contraindications: Whole plant.
Uterotropic Constituents: [Not identified.]
Described Activity: Emmenagogue.
References: 25, 100, 104

Vetiveria zizanoides (L.) Nash. Poaceae

Common Names: Vetiver
Parts Contraindications: Root, rhizome.
Uterotropic Constituents: [Not identified.]
Described Activity: Emmenagogue, abortifacient.
References: 25, 100

Vitex agnus-castus L. Verbenaceae

Common Names: Chaste berry
Parts Contraindications: Fruit.
Uterotropic Constituents: [Not identified.]

Described Activity: Emmenagogue.
References: 25, 100, 106, 107

Withania somnifera Dunal. Solanaceae

Common Names: Ashwagandha
Parts Contraindications: Fruit.
Uterotropic Constituents: Nicotine.
Described Activity: Emmenagogue, abortifacient.
References: 25, 100

Zanthoxylum spp.   Rutaceae

Common Names: Prickly ash
Parts Contraindications: Bark, berries.
Uterotropic Constituents: [Not identified.]
Described Activity: Emmenagogue.
References: 100, 103

Zingiber officinale Roscoe.   Zingiberaceae

Common Name: Ginger
Parts Contraindications: Dried root
Uterotropic Constituents: [Not identified.]
Described Activity: Emmenagogue, abortifacient.
References: 25, 102, 106

Ziziphus spp.   Rhamnaceae

Common Name: Ziziphus
Parts Contraindications: Seed, leaves, stem, bark.
Uterotropic Constituents: [Not identified.]
Described Activity: Uterine stimulant, emmenagogue, abortifacient.
References: 25, 10

References

1. R. Dreusback, Handbook of Poisoning, 8th ed., Lange Medical Publications, Los Altos, CA: 1974.

2. *Toxicants Occuring Naturally in Foods*, Committee on Food Protection, Food and Nutrition Board, National Research Council, National Academy of Sciences, Washington, D.C., 1973.

3. A.W. Kutts-Cheraux, *Naturae Medicina & Naturopathic Dispensatory*, Antioch Press, Yellow Springs, Ohio, 1953.

4. J. DiPalma, *Basic Pharmacology in Medicine*, McGraw-Hill Book Co., New York, N.Y., 1976.

5. D.G. Spoerke, Jr., *Herbal Medications*, Woodbridge Press Publishing Company, Santa Barbara, California, 1980.

6. W.H. Lewis and M.P.F. Elvin-Lewis, *Medical Botany*, John Wiley & Sons, New York, N.Y., 1977.

7. V.E. Tyler, L.R. Brady and J.E. Robbers, *Pharmacognosy*, 7th ed., Lea & Febiger, Philadelphia, Penn., 1976.

8. H.A. Stephens, *Poisonous Plants of the Central United States*, The Regents Press of Kansas, Lawrence, Kan., 1980.

9. H.W. Felter, *The Eclectic Materia Medica, Pharmacology and Therapeutics*, John K. Scudder, Cincinnati, Ohio, 1922.

10. F.E. Ellinwood, *American Materia Medica, Therapeutics and Pharmacognosy*, Ellingwood's Therapeutist, Chicago, Ill., 1919.

11. J.Parvati, *Hygieia, A Woman's Herbal*, Peter J. Levison Associates, San Francisco, CA, 1978.

12. W.R. James, *Know Your Poisonous Plants*, Naturegraph Publishers, Healdsburg, CA, 1973.

13. A. Gilman, L. Goodman and A. Goodman Gilman, *The Pharmacological Basis of Therapeutics*, 6th ed., MacMillan, New York, N.Y., 1980.

14. POISINDEX® System, Micromedex, Inc., Feb. 28, 1983, accessed at the Oregon Poison Control and Drug Information Center, Portland, Ore.

15. B. Bannister, et. al., "Cardiac Arrest Due to Liquorice-Induced Hypokalemia," *British Medical Journal*, September 17, 1977.

16. A. Cummings, "Severe Reduction of Serum Potassium Induced by Licorice," *Nursing Times*, March 11, 1976, pp. 367-370.

17. J. Sullivan et. al., "Pennyroyal Oil Poisoning and Hepatotoxicity," *JAMA*, Dec. 28, 1979, Vol. 242, No. 26, p. 2873-4.

18. A. Ballantyne et. al., "Herbal Cigarettes For Kicks," *British Medical Journal,* Dec. 25, 1976, pp. 1539-1540.

19. K.P. Mokhobe, "Herb Use and Necrodegenerative Hepatitis," *South African Medical Journal,* July 3, 1976, pp. 1096-1099.

20. R. Schoental, "Prevention or Cure? Use of Toxic Herbs and Geographic Pathology," *Tropical and Geographic Medicine,* 1972, pp. 194-198.

21. G.J. Kapadia et. al., "Carcinogenicity of Some Folk Medicinal Herbs in Rats," *Journal of the National Cancer Institute,* March, 1978, pp. 683-684.

22. G. Rosenstein et. al., "Podophyllum - A Dangerous Laxative," *Pediatrics,* March, 1976, pp. 419-421.

23. A.B. Segelman et. al., "Sassafras and Herb Tea; Potential Health Hazards," *Journal of the American Medical Association,* Aug. 2, 1976, p. 477.

24. I. Hirono et. al., "Carcinogenic Activity of Symphytum Officinale," *Journal of the National Cancer Institute,* September, 1978, pp. 865-868.

25. N. Farnsworth et. al., "Potential Value of Plants as Sources of New Antifertility Agents I," *Journal of Pharmaceutical Sciences,* April, 1975, pp. 535-596.

26. J. Brauchli et. al., "Pyrrolizidine Alkaloids from Symphytum Officinale, L. and Their Percutaneous Absorption in Rats," *Experientia,* Vol. 38, 1982, pp. 1085-1087.

27. C. Culvenor et. al., "Structure and Toxicity of the Alkaloids of Russian Comfery (Symphytum uplandicum Nyman), a Medicinal Herb and Item of Human Diet," *Experientia,* April 15, 1980, pp. 377-379.

28. C.L. Miranda et. al., "Dietary Copper Enhances Hepatotoxicity of Senecio Jacobaea in Rats," *Toxicants and Applied Pharmacology,* 1981, pp. 418-423.

29. J. Brauchli et. al., "Pyrrolizidine Alkaloids in Symphytum Officinale and Their Dermal Absorption in Rats," *Experientia,* 1981, pp. 667.

30. D. Nashel et al, "Acute Gouty Arthritis," *JAMA,* Jan. 1, 1982, Vol. 247, pp. 58-59.

31. G. Cordell et. al., "Experimental Antitumor Agents from Plants, 1974-76," *Lloydia,* Jan-Feb., 1977, Vol. 40, No. 1 pp. 1-44.

32. N.Z. Nyazema, "Poisoning Due to Traditional Remedies," *The Central Africa Journal of Medicine,* May, 1984, Vol. 30. No. 5, pp. 81-83.

33. K. A. Winship, "Toxicity of Comfrey," *Adverse Drug React. Toxicol. Rev.,* 1991, Vol. 10, No. 1, pp. 47-59.

34. J.L. Shupe et. al., "Teratogenic Plants," *Veterinary and Human Toxicology*, December, 1983, Vol. 25, No. 6, pp. 415-421.

35. M.M. Kliks, "Studies on the Traditional Herbal Anthelmintic Chenopodium Ambrodioides L.: Ethnopharmacological Evaluation and Clinical Trials," *Social Science and Medicine*, 1985, Vol. 21, No.8,pp. 879-886.

36. D. Crummett et. al., "Accidental Veratrum Viride Poisoning in Three 'Ramp' Foragers," *North Carolina Medical Journal*, September, 1985, Vol. 46, No. 9, pp. 469-471.

37. A. Sinha et. al., "Embryotoxicity of Betel Nuts in Mice," *Toxicology*, 1985, Vol. 37, No. 3-4, pp. 315-326.

38. M. Albert-Puleo, "Fennel and Anise as Estrogenic Agents," *Journal of Ethnopharmacology*, December, 1980, Vol. 2, No.4, pp. 337-344.

39. R.C. Scott & V.J. Seiwert, "The treatment of angina pectoris with pure crystalline khellin," *Ann. Int. Med.*, 1952, 36:1190-1197.

40. G.V. Anrep et al., "The coronary vasodilator action of khellin," *Am. Heart J.*, 1949, 37:531-542.

41. H.C. Grice et al., "Toxic Properties of Nordihydroguaiaretic Acid," *Fd. Cosmet. Toxicol.*, 1968, Vol. 6, pp. 155-161.

42. M. Katz and F. Saibil, "Herbal Hepatitis: Subacute Hepatic Necrosis Secondary to Chaparral Leaf," *J. Clin. Gastroenterol.*, 1990, Vol. 12, No. 2, pp. 203-206.

43. D.W. Gordon et al., "Chaparral Ingestion," *JAMA*, 1995, Vol. 273, No. 6, pp. 489-490.

44. A.Y. Smith et al., "Cystic Renal Cell Carcinoma and Acquired Renal Cystic Disease Associated with Consumption of Chaparral Tea: A Case Report, "*J. Urol.*, 1994, Vol. 152, pp. 2089-2091.

45. D. R. Shasky, "Contact Dermatitis from Larrea tridentata (Creosote Bush)," *J. Am. Acad. Dermatol.*, 1986, Vol. 15, No. 2, Pt. 1, pp. 302.

46. L.B. Willey et al., "Valerian Overdose: A Case Report," *Vet. Human Toxicol.*, 1995, Vol. 37, No. 4, pp. 364-365.

47. R.D. White et al., "Effects of Microsomal Enzyme Induction on the Toxicity of Pyrrolizidine (Senecio) Alkaloids," *J. Toxicol. Environ. Health*, 1983, Vol. 12, pp. 633-640.

48. R.J. Huxtable, "Herbal Teas and Toxins: Novel Aspects of Pyrrolizidine Poisoning in the United States," *Perspec. Biol. Med.*, 1980, Vol. 24, No. 1, pp. 1-14.

49. Z. Kowalewski et al., "Toxicity of berberine sulfate," *Acta Pol Pharm.*, 1975, Vol. 32, No. 1, pp. 113-120 (Chem. Abs. 83:91108u).

50. A.D. Turova et al., "Berberine," *Lekarslv. Sredstva iz Rast.*, 1962, pp. 303-307 (Chem. Abs. 58:763b).

51. F.T. Schein & C. Hanna, "The absorption, distribution and excretion of berberine," *Arch. intern. pharmacodynamie*, 1960, Vol. 124, pp. 317-325 (Chem. Abs. 54:14473e).

52. C.F. Poe and C.C. Johnson, "Toxicity of Hydrastine, Hydrastinine, and Sparteine," *Acta pharmacol. et toxicol.*, 1954, Vol. 10, pp. 338-346.

53. R.W. Fuller et al., "Bronchoconstriction response to inhaled capsaicin in humans," *J. Applied Physiol.*, 1985, Vol. 58, pp. 1080-1084.

54. B. Sandler & P. Aronson, "Yohimbine-induced Cutaneous Drug Eruption, Progressive Renal Failure, and Lupus-like Syndrome," *Urology*, 1993, Vol. 41, No. 4, pp. 343-345.

55. P.A.G.M. DeSmet & O.S.N.M. Smeets, "Potential risks of health food products containing yohimbe extracts," *Brit. Med. J.*, 1994, Vol. 309, pp. 958.

56. J.K Dawson et al., "Dangerous monoamine oxidase inhibitor interactions are still occurring in the 1990s," *J. Accident & Emerg. Med.*, 1995, Vol. 12, No. 1, pp. 49-51.

57. H. Lefebvre et al., "Pseudo-phaeochromocytoma after multiple drug interactions involving the selective monoamine oxidase inhibitor selegiline," *Clin. Endocrinol.*, 1995, Vol. 42, pp. 95-99.

58. A. Malchow-Moller et al., "Ephedrine as an anorectic: the story of the 'Elsinore pill'," *Internat. J. Obesity*, 1981, Vol. 5, pp. 183-187.

59. A. Jori et al., "Effect of Eucalyptol (1,8-cineole) on the Metabolism of Other Drugs in Rats and in Man," *Eur. J. Pharmacol.*, 1970, Vol. 9, pp. 362-366.

60. L.K.Wash & J.D. Bernard, "Licorice-induced Pseudoaldosteronism," *Am. J. Hosp. Pharm.*, 1975, Vol. 32, No. 1, pp. 73-74.

61. B.E. Barker et al., "Peripheral Blood Plasmacytosis Following Systemic Exposure to Phytolacca americana (Pokeweed)," *Pediatrics*, 1966, Vol. 38, No. 3, pp. 490-493.

62. C.H. Costello and C.L. Butler, "An Investigation of Piscidia Erythrina (Jamaica Dogwood)," *J. Am. Pharm. Assoc.*, 1948, Vol. 37, No. 3, pp. 89-97.

63. M.F.McFarland III & J. McFarland, "Accidental Ingestion of Podophyllum," *Clin. Toxicol.*, 1981, Vol. 18, No. 8, pp. 973-977.

64. D.E. Cassidy et al., "Podophyllum Toxicity: A Report of a Lethal Case and a Review of the Literature," *J. Toxicol. - Clin. Toxicol.*, 1982, Vol. 19, No. 1, pp. 35-44.

65. L.M Moher & S.A. Maurer, "Podophylum Toxicity: Case Report and Literature Review," *J. Fam. Pract.,* 1979, Vol. 9, No. 2, pp. 237-240.

66. A.A. Fisher, "Severe Systemic and Local Reactions to Topical Podophyllum Resin," *Cutis,* 1981, Vol. 28, pp. 233, 236, 242, 248, 266.

67. M.D. Karol et al., "Podophyllum: Suspected Teratogenicity from Topical Application," *Clin. Toxicol.,* 1980, Vol. 16, No. 3, pp. 283-286.

68. P. D'Adamo, "Chelidonium and Sanguinaria alkaloids as anti-HIV therapy," *J. Naturop. Med.,* 1992, Vol. 3, No. 1, pp. 31-34.

69. K.D. Rose et al., "Spontaneous Spinal Epidural Hematoma with Associated Platelet Dysfunction from Excessive Garlic Ingestion: A Case Report," *Neurosurgery,* 1990, Vol. 26, No. 5, pp. 880-882.

70. B.E. Burnham, "Garlic as a possible risk for postoperative bleeding," *Plastic & Reconstructive Surgery,* 1995, Vol. 95, No. 1, pp. 213.

71. J.F. Leonforte, "Contact dermatitis from Larrea (creosote bush)," *J. Am. Acad. Dermatol.,* Vol. 14, No. 2, Pt. 1, pp. 202-207.

72. R. Kaiser et al., "Analysis of Buchu Leaf Oil," *J. Agric. Food Chem.,* 1975, Vol. 23, No. 5, pp. 943-950.

73. H.S. Feldman & W.W.Youngken, "A Pharmacognostical Study of Buchu," *J. Am. Pharm. Assoc., Sci. Ed.,* 1944, Vol. 33, pp. 277-288.

74. S.D. Weisbord et al., "Poison on Line – Acute Renal Failure Caused by Oil of Wormwood Purchased through theInternet," *NEJM,* 1997, Vol. 337, No. 12, pp. 825-827.

75. A.I. Rudenko, "Pharmacology of androseme-leaf hemp," *Farmakol. i Toksikol,* 1953, Vol.16, No. 2, pp 36-40 (C.A. 47:12652I).

76. J. Desruelles et al., "Cardiotonic action of Apocynum cannabinum," *Therapie,* 1973, Vol. 28, No. 1, pp. 103-113 (C.A. 78:144015s).

77. N.K. Abubakirov & R.S. Yamatova, "New material sources for obtaining k-strophanthin," *Med. Prom. S.S.S.R.,* 1960, Vol. 14, No. 1, pp. 15-17 (C.A. 54:21643c).

78. S.M. Kupchan et al., "Tumor Inhibitors. IV. Apocannoside and Cymarin, the Cytotoxic Principles of Apocynum cannabinum L.," *J. Med. Chem.,* 1964, Vol. 7, pp 803-804.

79. J. Petricic, "Cardenolides from the roots of Asclepias tuberosa," *Arch. Pharm.,* 1966, Vol. 299, No. 12, pp. 1007-1011 (C.A. 66:76274a).

80. W.E. Hassan, Jr., & H.L. Reed, "Studies on Species of Asclepias. VI. Toxicology, Pathology, and Pharmacology," *J. Am. Pharm. Assoc., Sci. Ed.,* 1952, Vol. 41, pp. 298-300.

81. C.H. Costello & C.L. Butler, "The Estrogenic and Uterine-Stimulating

Activity of Asclepias tuberosa. A Preliminary Investigation," *J. Am. Pharm. Assoc., Sci. Ed.,* 1950, Vol. 39, pp. 233-237.

82. A. Panossian et al., "Plant adaptogens. II. Bryonia as an adaptogen," *Phytomed.,* 1997, Vol. 4, No. 1, pp. 85-99.

83. W. Hall, "The health risks of cannabis," *Austral. Fam. Phys.,* 1995, Vol. 24, No. 7, pp.1237-1240.

84. L. Rinaldi, "Marijuana: A Research Overview," *Alaska Med.,* 1994, Vol. 36, No. 2, pp. 107-113.

85. M. Albert-Puleo, "Mythobotany, pharmacology, and chemistry of thujone-containing plants and derivatives," 1978, *Econ. Bot.,* 32:65-74.

86. H.L. Osher et al., "Khellin in the treatment of angina pectoris," *N. Eng. J. Med.,* 1951, 244(9):315-321.

87. R.H. Rosenman et al., "Observations on the clinical use of visammin (khellin)," *JAMA,* 1950, 143(2):160-165.

88. E. Bombardelli et al., "Aesculus hippocastanum L.," *Fitoterapia,* 1996, 67(6):483-511.

89. H.C. Ferguson & L.D. Edwards, "A Pharmacological Study of a Crystalline Glycoside of Caulophyllum thalictroides," *J. Am. Pharm. Assoc.,* 1954, 43(1):16-21.

90. M.S. Flom et al., "Isolation and Characterization of Alkaloids from Caulophyllum thalictroides," *J. Pharm. Sci.,* 1967, 5(11):1515-1517.

91. R.B. Barlow & L.J. McLeod, "Some studies on cytisine and its methylated derivatives," *Br. J. Pharmac.,* 1969, 35:161-174.

92. J. Ulrichova et al., "Inhibition of Acetylcholinesterase Activity by some Isoquinoline Alkaloids," *Planta Med.,* 1983, 48:111-115.

93. D. Loew, "Phytotherapy in heart failure," *Phytomed.,* 1997, 4(3):267-271.

94. R.C. de Pasquale et al., "Composition and Biological Activity of the Fatty Seed Oil of Delphinium staphisagria - Note I," *Int. J. Crude Drug Res.,* 1985, 23(1):5-11.

95. J.D. Phillipson & C. Melville, "An investigation of the alkaloids of some British species of Equisetum," *J. Pharm. Pharmacol.,* 1960, 12:506-508.

96. J.A. Henderson et al., "The antithiamine action of Equisetum," *J. Am. Vet. Med. Assoc.,* 1952, 33:225-254.

97. T. Nakabayashi, "Thermostable antithiamine factor. II. Thiamine-decomposing substances of horsetail," *Vitamins,* 1957, 12:20-24.

98. A. Peggs & H. Bowen, "Inability to detect organo-silicon compounds in Equisetum and Thuja," *Phytochem.,* 1984, 23(8):1788-1789.

99. W.R. Phipps et al., "Effect of Flax Seed Ingestion on the Menstrual Cycle," *J. Clin. Endocrinol. Met.*, 1993, 77(5):1215-1219.

100. M. McGuffin et al. (eds.), *Botanical Safety Handbook*, CRC Press, Boca Raton, 1997.

101. P.A.G.M. De Smet et al. (eds.), *Adverse Effects of Herbal Drugs 2*, Springer-Verlag, Berlin, 1993.

102. P.A.G.M. De Smet et al. (eds.), *Adverse Effects of Herbal Drugs 3*, Springer-Verlag, Berlin, 1997.

103. M. Grieve, *A Modern Herbal*, Dover Publications, New York, 1971.

104. J. Lust, *The Herb Book*, Bantam Books, New York, 1974.

105. R. Tisserand & T. Balacs (eds.), *Essential Oil Safety*, Churchill Livingstone, Edinburgh, 1995

106. M. Blumenthal et al. (eds.), *The Complete German Commission E Monographs*, 1998, Integrative Medicine Communications, Boston, Mass.

107. T. Fleming et al. (eds.), *PDR for Herbal Medicines*, 1998, Medical Economics Co., Inc., Montvale, NJ.

108. T.Z. Woldemariam et al., "Analysis of aporphine and quinolizidine alkaloids from Caulophyllum thalictroides by densitometry and HPLC," *J. Pharmaceut. Biomed. Anal.*, 1997, 15:839-843.

109. J. Shuster, "Black Cohosh Root? Chasteberry Tree? Seizures!" *Hosp. Pharmacy*, 1996, 31(12):1553-1554.

110. W. Adolf & E. Hecker, "New irritant diterpene-esters from roots of Stillingia sylvatica L. (Euphorbiaceae)," *Tetrahedr. Lett.*, 1980, 21:2887-2890.

111. W.F. Clark et al., "Flaxseed: A potential treatment for lupus nephritis," *Kidney Internat.*, 1995, 48:475-480.

112. M.F. Cometa et al., "Acute Effect of Alkaloids from Hydrastis canadensis L. on Guinea-pig Ileum: Structure-Activity Relationships," *Phytother. Res.*, 1996, 10:S56-S58.

113. E.Roder et al., "Pyrrolizidinalkaloide aus Senecio aureus," *Planta Med.*, 1983, 49:57-59.

114. L.W. Smith & C.C.J. Culvenor, "Plant sources of hepatotoxic pyrrolizidine alkaloids," *J. Nat. Prod.*, 1981, 44(2):129-152.

115. G.A. Conway & J.C. Slocumb, "Plants used as abortifacients and emmenagogues by Spanish New Mexicans," *J. Ehnopharmacol.*, 1979, 1:241-261.

116. D.M. Fatovich, "Aconite: A Lethal Chinese Herb," *Ann. Emerg. Med.*, 1992, 21(3):309311.

117. Y-T. Tai et al., "Cardiotoxicity after accidental herb-induced aconite poisoning," *Lancet,* 1992, 340:1254-1256.

118. B. Tomlinson et al., "Herb-induced aconitine poisoning," *Lancet,* 1993, 341:370-371.

119. T.Y.K. Chan et al., Herb-induced Aconitine Poisoning Presenting As Tetraplegia," *Vet. Human Toxicol.,* 1994, 36(2):133-134.

120. S.B. Vohora et al., "Central nervous system studies on an ethanol extract of Acorus calamus rhizomes," *J. Ethnopharmacol.,* 1990, 28:53-62.

121. J.M. Pena et al., "Rapidly progressive interstitial renal fibrosis due to a chronic intake of a herb (Aristolochia pistolochia) infusion," *Nephrol. Dial. Transplant.,* 1996, 11:1359-1360.

122. M. Vanhaelen et al., "Identification of aristolochic acid in Chinese herbs," *Lancet,* 1994, 343:174.

123. M.-L. Vanherwegnem et al., "Rapidly progressive interstitial renal fibrosis in young women: association with slimming regimen including Chinese herbs," *Lancet,* 1993, 341:387-391.

124. B.M. Hausen et al., "The sensitizing capacity of Compositae plants," *Contact Derm.,* 1978, 4:3-10.

125. G. Willuhn et al., "Helenalin- and 11,13-Dihydrohelenalinester from Flowers of Arnica montana," *Planta Med.,* 1983, 49:226-231.

126. D.I. Macht & J.A. Black, "A pharmacological note on Baptisia tinctoria," *J. Am. Pharm. Assoc.,* 1927, 16(11):1056-1059.

127. H. Petershofer-Halbmayer et al., "Isolation of Hordenine ("Cactine") from Selenicereus grandiflorus (L.) Britt. & Rose and Selenicereus pteranthus (Link & Otto) Britt. & Rose," *Sci. Pharm.,* 1982, 50:29-34.

128. C.J. Barwell et al., "Deamination of hordenine by monoamine oxidase and its action on vasa deferentia of the rat," *J. Pharm. Pharmacol.,* 1989, 41:421-423.

129. V. Viranuvatti et al., "Effects of Capsicum Solution on Human Gastric Mucosa as Observed Gastroscopically," *Am J. Gastroenterol.,* 1972, 58:225-232.

130. H.G. Desai et al., "Effect of red chilli powder on DNA content of gastric aspirates," *Gut,* 1973, 14:974-976.

131. B.M. Myers et al., "Effect of Red Pepper and Black Pepper on the Stomach," *Am. J. Gastroenterol.,* 1987, 82(3):211-214.

132. T. K. Jones & B.M. Lawson, "Profound neonatal congestive heart failure caused by maternal consumption of blue cohosh herbal medication," *J. Pediatrics,* 1998, 132(3): 550-552.

133. C.C. Scott & K.K. Chen, "The pharmacological action of N-methylcytisine," *J. Pharm. Exp. Ther.*, 1943, 79:334-339.

134. O. Jonas & N. Smyth, "The use of syrup of ipecacuanha as a first-Aid measure in the management of accidental poisoning in the home," *Med. J. Austral.*, 1975, 1:534-535.

135. Anonymous, "Syrup of Ipecac Still Number One Choice," *Am. Pharm.*, 1981, NS21(2):46.

136. L. Guirola et al., "Acute Renal Failure from the Ingestion of Toxic Plants," *Vet. Hum. Toxicol.*, 1992, 34(6):548.

137. E. Genazzani & L. Sorrentino, "Vascular action of acteina: active constituent of Actaea racemosa L.," *Nature*, 1962, 194(4828):544-545.

138. D.I. Macht & H.M. Cook, "A pharmacological note on Cimicifuga," *J. Am. Pharm. Assoc.*, 1932, 21(4):324-330.

139. W. Siebert, "Percutaneous Absorption of Radioactively Tagged Camphor from Ointments," *Arzneim.- Forsch.*, 1964, 14:686-690.

140. E.C. Strain et al., "Caffeine Dependence Syndrome," *JAMA*, 1994, 272(13):1043-1048.

141. O.H. Drummer et al., "Three deaths from hemlock poisoning," *Med. J. Austral.*, 1995, 162:592-593.

142. J.H. Galloway, "Potentially hazardous compound in a herbal slimming remedy," *Lancet*, 1992, 340:179.

143. M.S. Lennard, "Genetic Polymorphism of Sparteine/Debrisoquine Oxidation: A Reappraisal," *Pharmacol. Toxicol.*, 1990, 67:273-283.

144. W. Klein-Schwatz & G.M. Oderda, "Jimsonweed Intoxication in Adolescents and Young Adults," *Am. J. Dis. Child.*,1984, 138:737-739.

145. J.P. Hanna et al., "Datura Delirium," *Clin. Neuropharm.*, 1992, 15(2):109-113.

146. L.H. Hassell & M.W. MacMillan, "Acute Anticholinergic Syndrome Following Ingestion of Angel's Trumpet Tea," *Haw. Med. J.*, 1995, 54:669-670.

147. G.S. Greene et al., "Ingestion of Angel's Trumpet: An Increasingly Common Source of Toxicity," *South. Med. J.*, 1996, 89(4):365-369.

148. P. Vlachos et al., "Lethal cardiac and renal failure due to Ecbalium elaterium (squirting cucumber)," *Clin. Toxicol.*, 1994, 32(6):737-738.

149. T. Powell et al., "Ma-Huang Strikes Again: Ephedrine Nephrolithiasis," *Am. J. Kidney Dis.*, 1998; 32(1):153-159.

150. Y. Tamura et al., "Effects of Glycyrrhetinic Acid and its Derivatives on

Δ^4-5α- and 5β-Reductase in Rat Liver," *Arzneim.-Forsch.*, 1979, 29:647-649.

151. T.J. Chamberlain, "Licorice Poisoning, Pseudoaldosteronism, and Heart Failure," *JAMA*, 1970, 213(8):1343.

152. M.T. Epstein et al., "Liquorice toxicity and the renin-angiotensin-aldosterone axis in man," *Br. Med. J.*, 1977, Jan. 22, pp. 209-210.

153. H. Kato et al., "3-Monoglucuronyl-Glycyrrhetinic Acid Is a Major Metabolite That Causes Licorice-Induced Pseudoaldosteronism," *J. Clin. Endocrinol. Metab.*, 1995, 80(6):1929-1933.

154. R.V. Farese Jr. et al., "Licorice-Induced Hypermineralocorticoidism," *New Engl. J. Med.*, 1991, 325(17):1223-1227.

155. G.J de Klerk et al., "Hypokalaemia and hypertension associated with use of liquorice flavoured chewing gum," *BMJ*, 1997, 314:731-732.

156. J.J. Chamberlain & I.Z. Abolnik, "Pulmonary Edema Following a Licorice Binge," *West. J. Med.*, 1997, 167:184-185.

157. S. Shintani et al., "Glycyrrhizin (Licorice)-Induced Hypokalemic Myopathy," *Eur. Neurol.*, 1992, 32:44-51.

158. M.T. Epstein et al., "Effect of eating liquorice on the rnein-angiotensis aldosterone axis in normal subjects," *Br. Med. J.*, 1977, Feb. 19, pp. 488-490.

159. J.A. Bakerink et al., "Multiple Organ Failure After Ingestion of Pennyroyal Oil From Herbal Tea in Two Infants," *Pediatr.*, 1996, 98(5):944-947.

160. I.B. Anderson et al., "Pennyroyal Toxicity: Measurement of Toxic Metabolite Levels in Two Cases and Review of the Literature," *Ann. Intern. Med.*, 1996, 124:726-734.

161. B.C. Smith & P.V. Desmond, "Acute hepatitis induced by ingestion of the herbal medication chaparral," *Aust. N. Z. J. Med.*, 1993, 23:526.

162. W.B. Batchelor et al., "Chaparral-induced hepatic injury," *Am. J. Gastroent.*, 1995, 90(5):831-833.

163. K.L. Grant et al., "Chaparral-Induced Hepatotoxicity," *Integrat. Med.*, 1998, 1(2):83-87.

164. U.T. Gutser et al., "Mode of antinociceptive and toxic action of alkaloids of Aconitum spec.," *Naun.-Schmied. Arch. Pharmacol.*, 1998, 357:39-48.

165. A. Ameri, "The effects of Aconitum alkaloids on the central nervous sytem," *Prog. Neurobiol.*, 1998, 56:211-235.

166. M. Depierreux et al., "Pathologic Aspects of a Newly Described Nephropathy Related to the Prolonged Use of Chinese Herbs," *Am. J. Kid. Dis.,* 1994, 24(2):172-180.

167. V. Monzani et al., "Acute Oleander Poisoning After a Selp-Prepared Tisane (Letter)," *Clin. Toxicol.,* 1997, 35(6):667-668.

168. A. Rezakhani & M. Maham, "Oleander Poisoning in Cattle of the Fars Province, Iran," *Vet. Hum. Toxicol.,* 1992, 34(6):549.

169. P. Thomas, "Oleander ingestion in a child," *Austral. Fam. Phys.,* 1998, 27(1/2):90-91.

170. G.S. Maritz et al., "Maternal nicotine exposure during pregnancy and development of emphysema-like damage in the offspring," *S. Afr. Med. J.,* 1993, 83:195-199.

171. R. Steldinger & W. Luck, "Half lives of nicotine in milk of smoking mother: implications for nursing," *J. Perinat. Med.,* 1988, 16:261-262.

172. V.J. Fontana, "Tobacco Hypersensitivity," *Ann. N.Y. Acad. Sci.,* 1960, 90:138-141.

173. T. Ferguson, *The Smoker's Book Of Health,* 1987, G.P. Putnam's Sons, New York.

174. J.L. Rios et al., "An Update Review of Saffron and its Active Constituents," *Phytother. Res.,* 1996, 10:189-193.

175. C.H. Linden et al., "Yohimbine: A New Street Drug," *Ann. Emerg. Med.,* 1985, 14:1002-1004.

176. S.A. Norton & P. Ruze, "Kava dermopathy," *J. Am. Acad. Dermatol.,* 1994, 31:89-97.

177. L. Schelosky et al., "Kava and dopamine antagonism," *J. Neurol. Neurosurg. Psychiatry,* 1995, 58(5):639-640.

178. Z.L.G. Stein, "Pokeweed-Induced Gastroenteritis," *Am J. Hosp. Pharm.,* 1979, 36:1303.

179. P.A. Kinamore et al., "Abrus and Ricinus Ingestion: Management of Three Cases," *Clin. Toxicol.,* 1980, 17(3):401-405.

180. P.J. Becci et al., "Short-term toxicity studies of sanguinarine and of two alkaloid extracts of Sanguinaria canadensis L.," *J. Toxicol. Environ. Health,* 1987, 20:199-208.

181. P. D'Adamo, "Chelidonium and Sanguinaria alkaloids as anti-HIV therapy," *J. Naturop. Med.,*1992, 3(1):31-34.

182. L.J. Ceha et al., "Anticholinergic toxicity from nightshade berry poisoning responsive to physostigmine," *J. Emerg. Med.,* 1997, 15(1):65-69.

183. C.G.M. Weston et al., "Veno-occlusive disease of the liver secondary to ingestion of comfrey," *Br. Med. J.,* 1987, 295:183.

184. P.M. Ridker et al., "Hepatic Venocclusive Disease Associated With the Consuption of Pyrrolizidine-Containing Dietary Supplements," *Gastroenterol.,* 1985, 88:1050-1054.

185. F.G. Miskelly & L.I. Goodyer, "Hepatic and pulmonary complicationsof herbal medicines," *Postgrad. Med. J.,* 1992, 68:935-936.

186. L.E. Sinn & J.F. Porterfield, "Lethal Taxine Poisoning from Yew Leaf Ingestion," *J. Forens. Sci.,* 1991, 36(2):599-601.

187. J. von der Werth & J.J. Murphy, "Cardiovascular toxicity associated with yew leaf ingestion," *Br. Heart J.,* 1994, 72:92-93.

188. E.P. Krenzelok et al., "Is the Yew Really Poisonous to You?" *Clin. Toxicol.,* 1998, 36(3):219-223.

189. J. Stebbing et al., "Deliberate self-harm using yew leaves (Taxus baccata)," *Br. J. Clin. Pract.,* 1995, 49(2).

190. K. Gelmon, "The taxoids: paclitaxel and docetaxel," *Lancet,* 1994, 344:1267-1272.

191. H.N. ElSohly et al., "Effect of Drying Taxus Needles on their Taxol Content: The Impact of Drying Intact Clippings," *Planta Med.,* 1995, 61:290-291.

192. D. Larrey et al., "Hepatitis after Germander (Teucrium chamaedrys) Administration: Another Instance of Herbal Medicine Hepatotoxicity," *Ann. Int. Med.,* 1992, 117:129-132.

193. L. Laliberte & J.-P. Villeneuve, "Hepatitis after the use of germancer, a herbal remedy," *Cn Med. Assoc. J.,* 1996, 154(11), 1689-1692.

194. N. Mostefa-Kara et al., "Lethal hepatitis after herbal tea," *Lancet,* 1992, 340:674.

195. D. Fau et al., "Diterpenoids From Germander, an Herbal Medicine, Induce Apoptosis in Isolated Rat Hepatocytes," *Gastroenterol.,* 1997, 113:1334-1346.

196. S. Foster, "Scullcap: an Herbal Enigma," *Business of Herbs,* 1996, May/June, pp. 14-16.

197. J.D. Phillipson & L.A. Anderson, "Herbal remedies used in sedative and antirheumatic preparations: Part 1," & "Part 2," *Pharmaceut. J.,* 1984, 233:80-82 & 111-115.

198. F.B. MacGregor et al., "Hepatotoxicity of herbal remedies," *Br. Med. J.,* 1989, 299:1156-1157.

199. L. Gealt et al., "Adult Respiratory Distress Syndrome After Smoke Inhalation From Burning Poison Ivy," *JAMA,* 1995, 274(4):358-359

200. M. Roulet et al., "Hepatic veno-occlusive disease in newborn infant of a woman drinking herbal tea," *J. Pediatr.*, 1988, 112(3):433-436.

201. I. Hirono et al., "Carcinogenic activity of coltsfoot, Tussilago farfara L.," *Gann*, 1976, 67:125-129.

202. W. Sperl et al., "Reversible hepatic veno-occlusive disease in an infant after consumption of pyrrolizidine-containing herbal tea," *Eur. J. Pediatr.*, 1995, 154:112-116.

203. A.M. Jaffe et al., "Poisoning due to ingestion of Veratrum viride (false hellebore)," *J. Emerg. Med.*, 1990, 8:161-167.

204. H.A. Spiller et al., "Retrospective Study of Mistletoe Ingestion," *Clin. Tox.*, 1996, 34(4):405-408.

205. J. Tibballs, "Clinical effects and management of eucalyptus oil ingestion in infants and yound children," *Med. J. Austral.*, 1995, 163:177-180.

206. T.E. Knight & B.M. Hausen, "Melaleuca oil (tea tree oil) dermatitis," *J. Am. Acad. Dermatol.*, 1994, 30:423-427.

207. A.C. de Groot & J.W. Weyland, "Systemic contact dermatitis from tea tree oil," *Cont. Derm.*, 1992, 27:279-280.

208. C. Elliott & A. Seawright, "Tea tree oil poisoning," *Med. J. Austral.*, 1993, 159:830-831.

209. M.A. Del Beccaro, "Melaleuca Oil Poisoning in a 17-Month-Old," *Ver. Hum. Toxicol.*, 1995, 37(6):557-558.

210. D. Villar et al., "Toxicity of melaleuca oil and related essential oils applied topically on dogs and cats," *Vet. Hum. Toxicol.*, 1994, 36(2):139-142.

211. E.C. Miller et al., "Structure-activity studies of the carcinogenicities in the mouse and rat of some naturally occurring and synthetic alkenylbenzene derivatives related to safrole and estragole," *Cancer Res.*, 1983, 43(3):1124-1134.

212. K. Randerath et al., "Phosphorus-32 post-labeling analysis of DNA adducts formed in the livers of animals treated with safrole, estragole and other naturally-occurring alkenylbenzenes," *Carcinogenesis*, 1984, 5(12):1613-1622.

213. M.S. Karawya et al., "Simultaneous TLC Separation of Khellin and Visnagin and Their Assay in Ammi visnaga Fruits, Extracts, and Formulations," *J. Pharm. Sci.*, 1970, 59(7):1025-1027.

214. O. Thastrup et al., "Coronary Vasodilatory , Spasmolytic and cAMP-Phosphodiesterase Inhibitory Properties of Dihydropyranocoumarins and Dihydrofuranocoumarisn," *Acta Pharmacol. et Toxicol.*, 1983, 52:246-253.

215. P. Khasigian et al., "Poisoning following oleander smoke inhalation," *J. Toxicol. Clin. Toxicol.*, 1998, 36(5):456-457.

216. K.A. Graeme et al., "Cardiotoxicity from ingestion of unprocessed Nerium oleander leaves treated with Fab fragments, *J. Toxicol. Clin. Toxicol.*, 1998, 36(5):457.

217. E. Schuetz, J. Adams, "Multi-system toxicity from intentional hellebore ingestion," *J. Toxicol. Clin. Toxicol.*, 1998, 36(5):454.

Index

A

T

Francis Brinker, N.D.

Francis Brinker, N.D., is a 1981 graduate of the National College of Naturopathic Medicine in Portland, Oregon. In addition, he completed the two year Postgraduate Studies Program in Botanical Medicine and taught Botanical Medicine there until 1985.

Dr. Brinker's undergraduate work includes a Bachelor of Science Degree in Human Biology from Kansas Newman College and a Bachelor of Arts Degree in Biology from the University of Kansas, Phi Beta Kappa.

He is a researcher of historic, scientific and medical literature on the subject of plant medicines and is currently providing the curriculum in botanical medicine for Dr. Andrew Weil's Program in Integrative Medicine at the University of Arizona College of Medicine.

In addition to numerous articles published in European and U.S. professional journals, Dr. Brinker is author of several books, including: *The Eclectic Dispensatory of Botanical Therapeutics, Vol. II*; *Formulas For Healthful Living*; and *Herb Contraindications and Drug Interactions*. In addition, he was a major contributor to *The Eclectic Dispensatory of Botanical Therapeutics, Vol.I*.

Books by Francis Brinker, N.D.

Available through Eclectic Medical Publications

◆

Herb Contraindications & Drug Interactions, *Second Edition*
Formulas for Healthful Living, *Second Edition*
The Eclectic Dispensatory of Botanical Therapeutics, Vol II.